TOWARD A NEW DIAGNOSTIC SYSTEM
FOR CHILD PSYCHOPATHOLOGY

Toward a New Diagnostic System for Child Psychopathology

Moving Beyond the DSM

PETER S. JENSEN
PENNY KNAPP
DAVID A. MRAZEK

THE GUILFORD PRESS
New York   London

© 2006 The Guilford Press
A Division of Guilford Publications, Inc.
72 Spring Street, New York, NY 10012
www.guilford.com

Printed in the United States of America

This book is printed on acid-free paper.

Last digit is print number: 9   8   7   6   5   4   3   2   1

Library of Congress Cataloging-in-Publication Data

Jensen, Peter S.
  Toward a new diagnostic system for child psychopathology : moving beyond the DSM / by Peter S. Jensen, Penny Knapp, David A. Mrazek.
      p. cm.
  Includes bibliographical references and index.
  ISBN 1-59385-251-7 (hardcover : alk. paper)
  1. Diagnostic and statistical manual of mental disorders. 2. Child psychopathology—Diagnosis. 3. Adolescent psychopathology—Diagnosis. 4. Child psychopathology—Classification. 5. Adolescent psychopathology—Classification.
  [DNLM: 1. Diagnostic and statistical manual of mental disorders. 2. Mental Disorders—diagnosis—Adolescent. 3. Mental Disorders—diagnosis—Child. 4. Adolescent Development. 5. Child Development. 6. Evolution. 7. Mental Disorders—classification—Adolescent. 8. Mental Disorders—classification—Child. WS 350 J538t 2006] I. Knapp, Penny. II. Mrazek, David. III. Title.
  RJ503.5.J45 2006
  618.92′89075—dc22

                                                                    2005027775

About the Authors

Peter S. Jensen, MD, is Director of the Center for the Advancement of Children's Mental Health, Ruane Professor of Child Psychiatry at the Columbia University College of Physicians and Surgeons, and Research Psychiatrist with the New York State Office of Mental Health and the New York State Psychiatric Institute. Before coming to Columbia University, he was Associate Director of Child and Adolescent Research at the National Institute of Mental Health (NIMH), where he served as an investigator on a number of NIMH multisite studies. Dr. Jensen currently directs several studies focused on implementing evidence-based assessment approaches and treatment guidelines in pediatric primary care, mental health, and school settings. He also serves on many editorial and scientific advisory boards, is the author of over 200 scientific articles and book chapters, and has written or coedited 12 books on children's mental health.

Penny Knapp, MD, is Medical Director at the State of California Department of Mental Health. She has recently retired from the faculty at the University of California, Davis, where she served as Chief of the Division of Child, Adolescent, and Family Psychiatry, and had extensive clinical and consulting activity, including pediatric consultation liaison and community consultation, in Sacramento County. Dr. Knapp is a member or fellow of several national organizations, including the American Academy of Child and Adolescent Psychiatry and the American Academy of Pediatrics. She has several dozen refereed publications and is a journal or book reviewer for several pediatric and child psychiatry journals.

David A. Mrazek, MD, is Chair of the Department of Psychiatry and Psychology at Mayo Clinic Rochester and Professor of Psychiatry and Pediatrics at Mayo Clinic College of Medicine. He currently serves as Director of the S. C. Johnson Genomics of Addictions Program and Director of the American Board of Psychiatry and Neurology. Before coming to Mayo Clinic, Dr. Mrazek served as Chair of Psychiatry and Behavioral Science at George Washington University School of Medicine, where he was the Leon Yochelson Professor of Psychiatry. He remains actively involved in psychiatric pharmacogenomic research, particularly therapeutic response to antidepressant medication. Dr. Mrazek is the author of over 200 publications.

Contributors

Markus Kruesi, MD, is Professor in the Department of Psychiatry and Behavioral Sciences at the Medical University of South Carolina. His research examines influences on aggression and disruptive behavior disorders (e.g., conduct disorder and attention-deficit/hyperactivity disorder) and uses magnetic resonance imaging to examine brain anatomy and function in conduct disorder. Dr. Kruesi is a coauthor of an emergency department protocol for adolescent suicide/homicide prevention that was rated effective by the Suicide Prevention Resource Center Registry of Evidence-Based Suicide Prevention Programs.

Cynthia R. Pfeffer, MD, is Professor of Psychiatry at Weill Medical College of Cornell University, where she is also Director of the Childhood Bereavement Program. She has studied extensively the risk for suicidal behavior in children and adolescents. Dr. Pfeffer's book *The Suicidal Child* (1986, Guilford Press) has been a mainstay in understanding suicidal behavior in youth.

Daniel S. Pine, MD, is Chief in the Section on Development and Affective Neuroscience and Chief of Child and Adolescent Research in the Mood and Anxiety Disorders Program of the National Institute of Mental Health. His research focuses on the biological and pharmacological aspects of mood, anxiety, and behavioral disorders in children and adolescents.

John Schowalter, MD, is the Albert J. Solnit Professor Emeritus of Child Psychiatry at the Yale Child Study Center, Yale University School of Medicine. He is past president of a number of national psychiatry organizations.

Theodore Shapiro, MD, is Professor Emeritus in the Department of Psychiatry at the Weill Medical College of Cornell University. He is author or editor of seven books and the author of more than 200 papers and scholarly chapters.

Laurence Steinberg, PhD, is Distinguished Professor and Laura H. Carnell Professor of Psychology at Temple University. His research focuses on a range of topics in the study of child and adolescent development, including parent–adolescent relationships, developmental psychopathology, adolescent employment, high school reform, and juvenile crime and justice.

Peter E. Tanguay, MD, is the Spafford Ackerly Endowed Professor of Child and Adolescent Psychiatry in the Department of Psychiatry and Behavioral Sciences at the University of Louisville School of Medicine. He is the author of numerous articles in leading journals on the subject of autism and has presented lectures and workshops in the United States, Europe, Japan, and China. Dr. Tanguay is also a member of the Group for the Advancement of Psychiatry and a fellow of the American College of Psychiatrists.

Preface

With the amazing new tools made possible by neuroscience and genetics, rapid strides have been made in the last few decades in understanding the linkages between brain and behavior, and specifically, mental disorders. How does this modern understanding of the brain and behavior relate to the theme of this volume? In fact, the modern era of diagnostic thinking was made possible only when Charles Darwin articulated his theory of natural selection 150 years ago. Until then, there had been but one way to understand human behavior—through the lens of good and evil. The theory of natural selection challenged the unitary biblical view that humans are unique creatures created by God in his image. Those poor souls who deviated from that perfect image were possessed by the devil. Harsh "treatment" to rid them of such possession logically followed. Darwin's new theory of the development of human behavior called for a new method of classification, one not oriented to demonology. Insanity became recognized as an illness. Neurasthenia, or neurotic illness, became differentiated from insanity, or psychotic illness. Next, Sigmund Freud, who supported the concept of neurasthenia as an advance in diagnostic thinking (even diagnosing himself as neurasthenic), split off two symptom clusters—anxiety and depression. That laid the groundwork for the modern neurobiological understanding of these two groups of disorders. For example, evolutionary theory has allowed us to observe how, over the course of time, the central nucleus of the amygdala became progressively smaller, while the basolateral nucleus and prefrontal cortex became larger and the connections between them elaborated. These changes in brain anatomy paralleled changes in human emotional states—the predominating fear of attack and physical harm characteristic of the primitive human condition became subordinated to newer affects such as shame or guilt (Kagan, 1998). Natural selection had shaped both structure and function. The key is the concept of adaptation.

Natural selection has a central organizing principle: A species will reproduce more rapidly than resources in the environment can support, so that over time, survival favors those among the species that develop the most adaptive characteristics. As an example, consider the evolution of human vision and its ramifications. For the solitary hunter on the Serengeti hundreds of thousands of years ago, sharpness of distance vision was adaptive, myopia clearly maladaptive. But by the Middle Ages, the random occurrence of myopia characterized the scholarly monk laboring over manuscripts by candlelight. Myopia was becoming adaptive for the larger society—beyond individual survival. The mutation survived because it had developed a future as an adaptive rather than maladaptive characteristic. Later, when reading became more than a specialized function of the scholarly monk, a universal need for general social and occupational adaptation, myopia became commonplace, now having a prevalence of 25%. But what happened next? Along with the heightened importance of literacy came an unexpected and unwanted side effect—a disorder of reading called dyslexia. It blossomed from a minor, largely unnoticed mutation to become a major social problem for a literate society. And that raises the most important question yet: Why does it survive if it is so maladaptive? The answer: Accompanying compensatory advantage gives it a reprieve. Consider the dyslexic medical student struggling with his or her phonological deficit and graduating in the bottom third of the class, but blossoming into an outstanding pathologist, radiologist, or surgeon because of compensatory three-dimensional perceptual skills. That's the reason. Maladaptive characteristics survive when they confer advantage as well as disadvantage. It's like the deadly sickling in Americans of African descent—protective against malaria in another continent, at another time.

Or consider the survival of bipolar illness in our society today. Some authors have noted its links to creativity in studies of artists, writers, and musicians (Andreasen & Glick, 1988; Jamison, 1994;

Nettle, 2004). In other words, if you are a creative genius, the odds are that there is bipolar susceptibility in your family beyond chance occurrence. Yes, it may be that other highly adaptive personality traits accompany certain Axis I mental illnesses and contribute to the survival of otherwise maladaptive conditions.

Consider also the application of this evolutionary model of adaptive/maladaptive symptoms to an all too familiar condition in our own society—conduct disorder. We find that it is much more complicated than simply aggressive behaviors that were adaptive in the Pleistocene age becoming maladaptive in the industrial age. Back then, in a primitive society in which a large number of individuals competed for a relatively small number of resources, when self-interest led to survival from predators, one can understand aggressive behavior as adaptive. But as the independent life of the individual hunter became less focused on self-preservation and gave way to communal or group living, not just for protection against predators, but for a greatly improved food supply, *control* over aggression and *effective* social interaction skills became the prized personality characteristics. Priorities had changed. Processing information to more accurately perceive others became a priority neurophysiological function, and where it developed, the species not only survived but thrived. At the same time, higher control centers were needed to interpret stimuli and mediate the aggressive response. The limbic system, including the amygdala, septal area, and hypothalamus, became involved in the inhibition of aggression.

Thus, the rapid evolution of a social-cognitive network formed by various centers in the brain (Harris, 1995) favored the development of the frontal and prefrontal lobes and the strategic deployment of aggressive strategies under more specified, refined conditions (see, e.g., Hawley, 2003). Furthermore, increasing human attachment behavior favored the expansion of the affective spectrum. Differentiating newer affects of not just fear, but also joy, anger, and sadness, became parallel developments of social advantage. The need for interconnections between these cognitive and affective behaviors accelerated the complexity of this system. Considering the consequences of the dysfunction of these regulatory systems, conduct disorder may be seen as a constellation of symptoms, reflecting not just deficits in social attachment behaviors (conduct) but also problems in the regulation of emotional and cognitive functions (anxiety and depression) resulting from neurophysiological perturbations of this complex regulatory system embedded in new environmental demands (Buss & Shackelford, 1997; Zoccolillo et al., 1992).

In this volume we outline the theoretical underpinnings of evolutionary theory as applied to some aspects of human behavior, particularly childhood psychopathology, where adaptation to one's environment is the crucial task of successful development. We consider the implications of this rethinking of our diagnostic terminologies in terms of etiology, prevention, and intervention. In an almost alternating fashion, as we have immersed ourselves in this literature in the service of this task, we have been enlightened, amused, skeptical, and astounded. We hope you enjoy this journey as much as we have.

PETER S. JENSEN, MD
PENNY KNAPP, MD
DAVID A. MRAZEK, MD

REFERENCES

Andreasen NC & Glick ID (1988) Bipolar affective disorder and creativity: Implications and clinical management. *Compr Psychiatry*, 29:207–217.

Buss DM & Shackelford TK (1997) Human aggression in evolutionary psychological perspective. *Clin Psychol Rev*, 17:605–619.

Harris JC (1995) *Developmental neuropsychiatry (Vol. 1: The fundamentals; Vol. 2: Assessment, diagnosis, and treatment of developmental disorders)*. New York: Oxford University Press.

Hawley PH (2003). Strategies of control, aggression, and morality in preschoolers: an evolutionary perspective. *J Exp Child Psychol*, 85:213–235.

Jamison KR (1994) *Touched with fire: Manic–depressive illness and the artistic temperament*. New York: Macmillan.

Kagan J (1998) *Three seductive ideas*. Cambridge, MA: Harvard University Press.

Nettle D (2004). Evolutionary origins of depression: a review and reformulation. *J Affective Disord*, 81:91–102.

Zoccolillo M, Pickles A, Quinton D, & Rutter M (1992) The outcome of childhood conduct disorder: Implications for defining adult personality disorder and conduct disorder. *Psychol Med*, 22:971–986.

Contents

CHAPTER 1

Introduction

PETER S. JENSEN *and* DAVID A. MRAZEK

Despite the apparent popularity and fairly widespread use of the fourth edition of the American Psychiatric Association's *Diagnostic and Statistical Manual of Mental Disorders* (DSM-IV), there remain lingering concerns among clinicians and the general public about the applicability of "mental disorder" status to many conditions and situations currently listed in this nomenclature. Particularly among persons who work with children, concerns have been raised that many of the difficulties experienced by children reflect problems in adaptation, the impact of adverse experiences, or a mismatch between the child's developmental needs and the resources available in the environment.

The apparent reification and attendant expansion of diagnostic categories seems increasingly implausible, as current evidence suggests that the diagnostic categories represent syndromes with heterogenous etiologies. Furthermore, neuroscience research has provided evidence that early environmental experiences have significant impact on structural and functional aspects of cortical development, neuronal activity, and organization. Although diagnostic nomenclature "drives" most insurance and reimbursement-related decision making, much of the public finds the language difficult to comprehend and counterintuitive. Moreover, risk factor research suggests that most risk factors are nonspecific and are similarly related to all disorders (Hann & Borek, 2001). Likewise, treatments are not diagnosis-specific, but symptom-specific. Diagnosis per se often has little impact on specific treatments selected for children, and treatment is instead designed on the basis of the child's symptom profile and nature of his or her impairments. Even in the major public settings where many children's services are delivered (e.g., the schools), the diagnostic nomenclatures are generally avoided and treatments are based on specific areas of functional impairment.

So how did this state of affairs come about? Prior to the introduction of the more recent versions of the DSM (versions III, III-R, IV, and IV-TR), cases of mental disorder were defined principally as a function of decades of amalgamated clinical experience in identifying clusters of commonly occurring syndromes. In one sense, cases were "cases" by virtue of their presentation for clinical care (Cantwell, 1996). Yet in times of shrinking resources, simple presentation for care to a clinical setting is not an adequate definition of disorder, as some persons presenting to clinical settings may in fact not require substantive clinical treatment resources. Moreover, some persons not seeking care may in fact need and benefit from mental health treatments. With the advent of these more rigorously descriptive diagnostic nomenclatures, mental disorder "caseness" determination became feasible within nonclinical settings (e.g., epidemiological studies), offering the possibility for replicable research exploring mental disorders' risk and protective factors, course, and outcome, in ways that prior to that point were difficult or impossible. From policy and public health vantage points, determination of unmet needs for care came within reach. Obviously, in addition to the scientific need to know what constitutes a "mental disorder," public health approaches to mental illness require that persons in need of care (whether in the treatment system or not) be reliably determined.

Of note, these two goals—the reliable identification of valid syndromes, such that research can identify their causes, consequences, and effective treatments, and the determination of when a person's symptoms are such that public resources should be expended to render prevention and treatment services—were fused with the introduction of DSM-III. Prior to that time, researchers' objectives for a reliable diagnostic system were met via approaches such as the Washington University Research Diagnostic Criteria, whereas other, less stringent systems as embodied in the DSM-II specifically for children, such as the Group for the Advancement of Psychiatry (GAP) system, allowed clinicians considerable leeway in determining when a case was a case. Fusion of both objectives within DSM-III and beyond has had substantial ramifications for good and ill, as will be discussed in chapters that follow.

SO WHY THIS VOLUME?

In view of the considerable questions surrounding how to best determine the "caseness" of children's mental disorders for both of the aforementioned purposes, our goal with this volume is to identify and discuss the most important issues relevant to defining mental disorder in clinical practice, research, and policy and to offer alternative approaches that we find better fit the actual phenomena—the developing child emerging in the context of complex environments, shaping and being shaped by his or her environments, and doing the best he or she can to fit within the particular niche that nature has provided.

In this first chapter, we set the stage for later chapters by reviewing problems in current diagnostic systems. We then introduce evolutionary and adaptational models, showing their power and usefulness in thinking both developmentally and contextually about given syndromes as well as specific cases. In the second chapter, we discuss what skilled clinicians actually do, and how they use a quite different process in coming to a sensible formulation of a patient's problem, beyond simple diagnosis. Chapter 3 describes temperament and development from an adaptational and evolutionary perspective. Discussion of specific syndromes/disorders within these alternative approaches then follows, with Chapters 4–9 on anxiety, depression, attention-deficit/hyperactivity disorder (ADHD), conduct disorder, stress disorders, autism, and developmental disorders. In the 10th and final chapter, we discuss implications for evaluation and treatment offered by our conceptual approach, we describe how treatments are better defined and more easily understood when couched within adaptational models, and we close with recommendations for research and clinical practice.

EVOLUTIONARY AND ADAPTATIONAL APPROACHES TO UNDERSTANDING MENTAL HEALTH AND ILLNESS

Given what we know about early plasticity and children's responsiveness to environmental modifications, the counterintuitive and theoretical nature of current nosologic systems, alternative ways to understand these phenomena of childhood behavioral and emotional disturbances are needed. One worthy candidate is biological systems theory—natural selection has shaped the tools we have, and much of the work of the mind may be seen as the products of mental organs whose purpose is to enhance adaptation. From this perspective, humans can be viewed as "adaptation machines," intended to fit to a range of environments, all within what evolutionary biologists term the "environment of evolutionary adaptedness" (EEA). Viewed from this perspective, some of our so-called mental disorders may be thought to reflect different levels of interaction between brain and environment, and the consolidation of these interactions over time in stressful environments much different in nature from their ancestral precursors (Garruto, Little & Weitz, 2004).

Interestingly, despite the commonsense nature of this approach and its relevance to much of medicine and biology, to date there has been little application of biological systems theory and evolutionary models to our understanding, clinical modeling, and research approaches to mental health and illness (Nettle, 2004).

PSYCHOPATHOLOGY AND ADAPTATION

Central to evolutionary and adaptationist approaches to organizing the mass of data from the behavioral, cognitive, and clinical psychopathology sciences is to consider fully the issues of adaptation: According to Mayr (2001), "the adaptationist question, 'What is the function of a given structure or organ?' has been for centuries the basis for every advance in physiology.'" Although behavioral researchers have generally shied away from them, theories of adaptive function are an indispensable methodologic tool. Along this line, Mayr (1980) has argued that "a program's structure depends more upon the computational problems that have to be solved than upon the particular hardware in which the solutions are implemented." In other words, knowing *what* and *why* places strong constraints on theories of *how*. Although not everything in the design of organisms is the product of selection, all complex functional organization arguably is. Thus, regarding the brain's major outputs (thoughts, feelings, behaviors) as specific functions greatly shaped by selective processes offers the possibility to organize and understand much human behavior within the rubric of problem-solving, information-processing systems. In Mayr's explanatory approach, form follows function:

1. Information-processing systems are designed to solve problems.
2. These systems solve problems by virtue of their structure.
3. Hence, to explain the structure of a device, you need to know what problem(s) it was designed to solve and why it was designed to solve this particular problem and not some other one.

Furthermore, one might then proceed from the third point to ask, "What is the adaptive problem?" and "What information would have been available in ancestral environments for solving the problem?"

Adaptive problems posed by social life are substantial. According to Cosmides and Tooby (1997), most of these problems are characterized by strict evolvability constraints and can be satisfied only by cognitive programs specialized for reasoning about the social world. This suggests that our mental architecture contains a large faculty of social-cognitive capacities. Cosmides and Tooby suggest that tasks are usually solved by complex cognitive machinery that is highly specialized. For example, they and others suggest the existence of domain-specific adaptive specializations with a certain readiness to attend to certain types of cues and respond to certain stimuli but not others. Consider, for example, the observations of Marks and Nesse (1994) about the human propensity to develop snake and spider phobias, but insufficient readiness to show appropriate fearfulness of guns or cars, or high-cholesterol foods, which are, in fact, much more relevant health hazards in our modern day. Another example is the well-known infant's capacity and preference for observation of the human face versus other, novel stimuli.

RETHINKING PSYCHIATRIC ILLNESSES

Psychiatric disorders are the result of not just environmental factors, nor of biological factors exclusively. Rather, "disorders" are the result of the progressive development of the brain as it unfolds within the constraints of the genomic map and the particular environmental circumstances and context of a given organism. An evolutionary biological perspective on psychiatric disorders seems to implicitly support the notion of noncategorical approaches, inasmuch as evolutionary theory presupposes an adaptive fit, or "fine-tuning" of the organism's responses to subtle but meaningful environmental differences. Yet at some points, development and adaptation can be discontinuous, as the particular lack of fit between an organism and a given environment may overwhelm the organism's adaptive responses and qualitatively different systems are brought in line in an unsuccessful attempt to compensate (e.g., see Amiel-Tison et al., 2004). At times, the actions and interactions of "odd" risk factors (e.g., where an expected effect is not seen if accompanied by another factor) and the presence of serendipitously discovered interactions may provide clues to these kinds of qualitatively different mechanisms or discontinuous functions.

From this perspective, a number of mechanisms may be invoked to explain the presence and persistence of "psychopathology" in the gene pool, as well as its existence in any given member in the population:

- Genetic drift (mutation) with no natural selection; that is, the trait has no bearing on reproductive success.
- Correlated consequences. The maladaptive trait is correlated with some other trait(s) that are themselves adaptive. The maladaptive trait is part of a package that has some evolved value. Depression may be correlated with ability to form pair-bonds, for example.
- Environmental change. A trait that was adaptive in our ancestral environment is no longer adaptive because of environmental change. A corollary of this is that the psychopathology "cut-point" on a distribution has shifted over time owing to changes in the environment. ADHD is a nice example.
- Selection without adaptation (Gould & Lewontin, 1978). The maladaptive trait is correlated with increased fecundity. Males

with antisocial personality disorder can more easily persuade females to bear their offspring.

- The trait is the result of an evolved plasticity and susceptibility to (early) environmental influence, coupled with an environment that has facilitated the development of the trait.
- Heterozygote advantage. According to this model, persons with one allele of a given recessive gene are selected, because the single copy conveys some protection (e.g., Tay–Sachs, tuberculosis, cystic fibrosis, cholera, sickle cell anemia, malaria). Could single copies of certain genes lead to higher energy, productivity, creativity, with only the homozygous individuals significantly adversely affected?

Given the presence in the gene pool of susceptibility factors (through any of the mechanisms noted earlier), how might behavioral ecological and evolutionary perspectives view the presence of a disorder in a specific organism at any point in time? We suggest a number of possibilities.

- First, the human organism and its systems are under stress. While attempting to maintain homeostasis and equilibrium, the organism is stretched beyond what it/he/she evolved to be able to do. In such a scenario, "disorder" reflects the organism's attempts to maintain homeostasis in an overtaxed, failing system. Posttraumatic stress disorder might reflect such processes.
- Second, the presence of disorder may reflect the interaction of the aforementioned process with the constitution of an organism who is susceptible by virtue of less adaptation equipment (e.g., a person "genetically" or "epigenetically" prone to conduct disorder or depression).
- Third, arguably some instances of "disorders" may reflect processes whereby the organism has been shaped by early environment to fit that environment, and then is thrust into another in a larger societal context where the shaped behaviors are nonadaptive (e.g., some cases of conduct disorder may fit this prototype). Similarly, mental health professionals working with aborigines in Australia have reported that aboriginal children have a very active, scanning-type attention and in traditional environments might meet criteria for ADHD. Those attempting to teach these children in traditional classroom environments have found that they must go to extraordinary

lengths to keep the children's attention and have to break activities into many small segments. Potentially, as the organism becomes less malleable (plastic) over time, he or she may be at more risk to become dysfunctional, depending on the ability of the organism to adapt to new circumstances and the degree of change in the circumstances and new environments. Various terms to describe the increased specification and individualization of capacities have been used, such as the "canalization" of development and, relatedly, the "orthogenetic hypothesis."

• Fourth, it is quite plausible that the organism's "adaptation equipment" simply does not work according to the demands of the EEA, (e.g., autism, schizophrenia). In other words, despite a range of average expectable environments, major deficits in functioning may be apparent, presumably as a function of abnormal brain development, organization, and structure.

• Fifth, in a developmental twist of the fourth possibility, it is conceivable that the organism has an underlying developmental disturbance, and as the rest of organism attempts to adjust, the disorder becomes more apparent over time (e.g., schizophrenia as a disorder of abnormal reinervation). In other words, the external manifestations of the "disease" are organismic attempts to adjust or compensate.

• Sixth and last, there may be a progressive failure of the organism's ability to modulate an adaptive ability—in other words, an adaptive ability may have gone awry. For example, a certain amount of checking and cleaning may be quite adaptive, and a prominent part of human functions, especially around the time of childbirth. But if in the range of human variation this natural function is "set too high," extreme behaviors of this nature may become impairing and dysfunctional (Leckman & Mayes, 1998).

It is important to note that great care and critical thought are needed when applying evolutionary accounts to human behavior (Gould & Lewontin, 1978). Clearly, many behaviors may never be and might never have been adaptive, whatever the environmental circumstances. For example, it is difficult to conceive of circumstances where severe mental retardation or full-blown autism would convey some evolutionary advantage. In addition, some traits are poor objects of evolutionary explanation because they never served an evolutionary function, no longer serve a function, are components of an adaptation that is best analyzed at another level, are manifestations of phylogenetic constraints, or result from fixation of mutations by genetic drift.

Naive oversimplifications of selection processes must be avoided. It is highly unlikely that natural selection shaped fixed patterns of response. More likely is that natural selection has shaped propensities to establish and maintain certain conditioned avoidance reactions, and capacities to adjust these to the current environment.

Despite the attractiveness of some evolutionary accounts, there are difficulties in "proving" such models and/or building empirical support. Thus, such models may be useful only to the extent that they provide new insights or lead to new clinical or research questions, with potential eventual relevance to practice and/or policy. Taking up this challenge, in the chapters that follow, we attempt to apply current thinking based on evolutionary, developmental, and neuroscientific principles to specific disorders.

REFERENCES

Amiel-Tison C, Cabrol D, Denver R, Jarreau PH, Papiernik E, & Piazza PV (2004) Fetal adaptation to stress: Part II. Evolutionary aspects; stress-induced hippocampal damage; long-term effects on behavior; consequences on adult health. *Early Hum Dev*, 78:81–94.

Cantwell DP (1996) Classification of child and adolescent psychopathology. *J Child Psychol Psychiatry Allied Disciplines*, 37:3–12.

Cosmides J & Tooby J (1997) Dissecting the computational architecture of social inference mechanisms. *Ciba Found Symp*, 208:132–161.

Garruto RM, Little MA, & Weitz CA (2004) Environmental stress and adaptational responses: Consequences for human health outcomes. *Coll Antropol*, 28:509–540.

Gould SJ & Lewontin RC (1978) The spandrels of San Marco and the Panglossian Paradigm: A critique of the Adaptationist Programme. *Proc R Soc London*, 205:581–598.

Hann DM & Borek NT (Eds.) (2001) *Taking stock of risk factors for child/ youth externalizing behavior problems. (NIH Publication No. 02-4938).* Washington, DC: U.S. Government Printing Office.

Leckman JF & Mayes LC (1998) Understanding developmental psychopathology: How useful are evolutionary accounts? *J Am Acad Child Adolesc Psychiatry*, 37:1011–1021.

Marks IM & Nesse RM (1994) Fear and fitness: An evolutionary analysis of anxiety disorders. *Ethol Sociobiol*, 15:247–261.

Mayr E (1980) *The evolutionary synthesis: Perspectives on the unification of biology.* Cambridge, MA: Harvard University Press.

Mayr E (2001) *What evolution is.* New York: Basic Books.

Nettle D (2004) Evolutionary origins of depression: A review and reformulation. *Affective Disord*, 81:91–102.

CHAPTER 2

Research and Clinical Perspectives in Defining and Assessing Mental Disorders in Children and Adolescents

PETER S. JENSEN *and* DAVID A. MRAZEK

Since the classic contribution of Robins and Guze (1970), a commonly accepted approach to validating a given set of commonly occurring symptoms has been by demonstration; that is, the purported disorder can be shown to demonstrate a number of distinguishing characteristics. More recently this approach has been modified by Cantwell (1996), with validation of a putative disorder assumed to be accomplished if the candidate disorder can be shown to be discriminable from other disordered states (as well as normal functioning) by any or all of the following: clinical descriptors (apart from the symptoms of the disorder itself), psychosocial factors, demographic factors, biological factors, family genetic factors, family environmental factors, natural history, and response to treatment.

Despite the potential usefulness of this approach, most of our current diagnoses, as implemented within the fourth edition of the American Psychiatric Association's *Diagnostic and Statistical Manual* (DSM-IV), fall short of this ideal validation standard. For example, at the 1998 National Institutes of Health (NIH) Consensus Development Conference on ADHD (attention-deficit/hyperactivity disorder) the conference panelists concluded that there was *some* evidence of validity for the diagnosis of ADHD, in terms of a number of these validating characteristics (principally family genetic factors, natural history, and response to treatment), but in other areas (e.g., specific biological factors) evidence to date is lacking. Notably, Werry and colleagues (1987) conducted a careful comparison of these criteria among ADHD, conduct disorders, and anxiety disorders, finding little support for the discrimination of even these major syndromes among themselves. Despite the lack of validating evidence concerning our major classification schemas for many of the most common childhood mental disorders, the greater psychiatric research and clinical communities have instead taken most of our major disorder categories at face value (if only by default), or when conducting comparisons have confined them principally to comparisons of cases of disorder with normal controls, or comorbid versus noncomorbid cases (see, e.g., Jensen et al., 2002).

This situation is not unique to childhood disorders, but bedevils most DSM-IV-defined adult conditions as well. Thus, if one asks, does the current DSM "carve nature at its joints," the research literature principally answers in the negative. For example, in a study of the diagnostic criteria for depression using a sample of monozygotic and dizygotic twins, Kendler and Gardner (1998) examined the diagnostic criteria for number of symptoms, severity, and duration, finding that number of symptoms and severity (but not duration) predicted increased likelihood of subsequent episodes in the index case and the twin. However, there was no natural cut-point at four symptoms: even persons with fewer than five symptoms, as well as having less severe symptoms (below diagnostic threshold), were at greater risk for subsequent episodes of depression, both in the index case and in the twin. These findings suggested that even subthreshold depressive symptoms reveal the same underlying diathesis. In addition, no support was found for the requirement of 2 weeks' duration or some threshold of clinical severity. Thus, major depressive disorder appeared to be a diagnostic convention imposed on a continuum of depressive symptoms of varying severity, impairment, and duration. Similar findings have been found in the area of genetic studies of ADHD, where heritability analyses of full syndrome versus subthreshold symptom states suggested that the condition likely reflected a continuum versus an all-or-none, present–absent psycho-pathological state (Levy et al., 1997; Rasmussen et al., 2002).

DISORDER DEFINITION VERSUS
MEDICAL NECESSITY

Despite the well-specified criteria in the most recent versions of the DSM, it has become clear that different methods of determining the presence or absence of these criteria can have a profound impact on supposed prevalence. Thus, Boyle and colleagues (1996) have found that differing strategies, such as using a three-point checklist that inquires about the presence of symptoms on a frequency scale (0 = never, 1 = sometimes, 2 = often), a structured diagnostic interview, or statistical strategies that require a range of deviation from the norm, result in dramatic (120-fold) differences in prevalence (Boyle et al., 1996), as well as substantial differences in test–retest reliability, interrater reliability, and comorbidity. Thus, a range of methodologic issues can contribute to substantial variations in mental disorder caseness determination, including the type of measurement instrument, the nature of the informant (e.g., parent, teacher, child), the scoring system, the chosen cutoffs for symptom levels, and symptom severity. As a result, it has been generally concluded that the presence of the diagnostic criteria alone provides insufficient grounds for determining "when a case is a case" (Boyle et al., 1996).

Even when one determines the presence or absence of symptoms using the most rigorous methods, such as face-to-face diagnostic interviews, variations in mental disorder definition are marked, based on ancillary determinations that are not necessarily part of the DSM criteria. Thus, Angold and colleagues (1999) examined the impact of various definitions of *impairment* on rates of serious emotional disturbance, after first requiring that all children considered meet all DSM symptomatic criteria. Using five different definitions of impairment in their study, Angold and colleagues compared children with neither impairment nor a diagnosis, those with no full-blown disorder but with impairment, those with disorder but no impairment, and those with both. Even among those who met both symptom and more stringent impairment criteria, only 59% of these families reported having a "need for services," and fewer still (19%) of those meeting diagnostic criteria with levels of impairment as specified within the DSM-IV criteria were reported as having any need for services. Even with the most stringent impairment criteria, two-thirds of those with a defined serious emotional disturbance were not being served.

In an important sense, then, clinicians', researchers', and clinical policymakers' wishes for precision in the determination of mental disorder have been thwarted by the fact that there are major differences in reported prevalence rates in state-of-the-art studies intended to address this major question, such as the dramatic (more than threefold in some instances) differences in prevalence rates in the National Institute of Mental Health (NIMH) Epidemiologic Catchment Area study (ECA) and the National Comorbidity Survey (NCS) (Regier et al., 1998).

To address this problem, particularly because the differences in prevalence rates occur principally around more commonly occurring syndromes, and to avoid future such controversies that may incite suspicion or ridicule by opponents of parity for mental health care, Regier and colleagues (1998) recommend that only the more severe disorders with public policy implications be examined in future epidemiological studies. Recounting the differences between epidemiological survey-identified "cases" and clinically identified cases, they note that community-defined cases are not likely to be as severe and may, in fact, be transient, "nonpathologic homoeostatic responses." Yet as noted by Spitzer (1998), both the ECA and NCS accounts of disorders are similarly related to external validators of psychopathology, suggesting that both measured something valid. Thus, Spitzer cautions that researchers should not confuse the identification of valid syndromes with the need for treatment, either by their avoiding such studies altogether, or by requiring extraordinary levels of impairment to justify determination of mental disorder, just to appease a skeptical public when such conditions are indeed valid disorders.

This situation may not differ much from other areas of medicine—thus, if respiratory disease specialists conducted surveys of the nationwide prevalence of "respiratory illness," inclusion of conditions ranging from upper respiratory illness to chronic obstructive pulmonary disease, asthma, and mild upper respiratory illnesses would likely result in nearly 100% rates of "disorder." Turning the question on its head, Spitzer asks why we need such studies when other areas of medicine do not?

Frances (1998) suggests that there are indeed clear limitations in defining clinical cases within epidemiological studies, in part because the DSMs fail to provide clear boundaries between normality and psychopathology, and because the concepts of *clinical significance* and *medical necessity* are difficult to operationalize and beyond the capability of lay interviewers. In addition, given the inherent variability in rates of disorder across settings, times, and cultures, epidemiological studies may overestimate the prevalence and/or significance of milder conditions.

Inspection of the differences between the NCS and ECA national surveys is instructive and suggests that sizable variations in reporting rates occur simply as a function of the placement of "stem questions" (those questions asked of all interviewees in a highly structured interview where many in-depth questions are skipped if the answer to a stem question is negative) at the beginning of the interview or instead spread throughout each of the diagnostic sections. Regardless, the different public presentations of rates of mental disorder may indeed be confusing and can make it difficult to build an incremental knowledge base for scientific or policy purposes.

Some commentators have suggested that the problem lies not so much within the survey methods as with the conceptual underpinnings of what constitutes "mental disorders." For example, Wakefield (1992) has noted that the philosophical underpinnings of the DSMs' accounts of disorder are structurally flawed and has argued that other accounts, such as "harmful dysfunction," better describe a valid, conceptually sound construct of disorder that has the dual requirements of some sort of "biological dysfunction" and cultural and contextual appraisal (see Kirk & Hsieh, 2004; Wakefield et al., 2002) of impairment ("harm") to warrant the determination of "true" mental disorder status. Yet this definition too is problematic, suffering from the tautological definition of dysfunction as a "biological system not behaving as it was designed to do" (from an evolutionary perspective). In addition, such a definition is further problematic because there are, as yet, no well-established biological indicators of dysfunction for any of the child mental disorders, and such definitions invoke anachronistic notions of some hard-and-fast lines between so-called biological and sociocultural factors (Nelson & Bloom, 1997; Wallace, 1994).

To avoid the conceptual muddles noted earlier in answering the question, "When is a case a case?", the first issue that must be addressed is "a case for what purpose?" For example, Sonuga-Barke (1998) notes that in order to distinguish between various definitions of disorder, one must clarify whether one wishes to define mental disorder for purposes of the clinical utility of such a definition (the "pragmatic view") or construct validity (the ontologic view). Although the ultimate goal of classification is *usefulness* (Frances, 1998), as Eisenberg (1995) has noted, there are many "usefulnesses." What works for researchers to define some presumably homogenous entity (i.e., the attempt to "carve nature at its joints") may not work well for clinicians and policymakers, who often wish to know "who needs care?"

One potential route out of such impasses in setting objectives has been described by Zarin and Earls (1993), who have recommended that methods of decision analysis be applied to such issues. They note that the essential components of diagnostic decision making—choice of external validator, choice of discriminator, and choice of cutoff scores—might be implemented very differently, depending on whether the clinician/investigator's objectives are to (1) determine which children need psychiatric care, where overall assessments of disability are most relevant; (2) determine what clinicians do in real-world practice (i.e., services research, which often varies from the "ideal-world" practice); and (3) determine which children constitute valid cases of a specific disorder, for purposes of research into etiology, genetic factors, treatment response, and likelihood of persistence/recurrence.

Thus, "caseness for what purpose" is the relevant question, and it must be appreciated that any cutoff or disciminator will result in some false negatives and false positives. The choice of cutoffs will often depend on the relative costs of false negatives versus false positives, vis-à-vis the clinical or research objectives.

PROBLEMS IN DEFINING CASENESS OF MENTAL DISORDER

Inspection of the range of challenges in determining mental disorder caseness in children and adolescents suggests that many of these issues are not unique to children and adolescents per se, but are shared with the caseness challenges that are part and parcel of adult studies (as noted earlier), as well as with other aspects of medicine. These issues include questions concerning categorical versus dimensional distinctions, choice of cutoffs, distinguishing diagnosis from the need for treatment, cultural factors affecting diagnosis and impairment, and the role of context. However, a set of somewhat unique items appears to be of relatively greater import in defining mental disorder within child and adolescent populations, namely, the role of children's caretaking environments vis-à-vis mental disorder, determining how to combine information from multiple informants, and special considerations that must be taken into account with young persons, principally as a function of the rapid rates of change occurring within their biological, psychological, and social capacities. We discuss these special challenges in the following sections, beginning first with those issues common to children and adults.

Categories or Dimensions?

A major conceptual consideration underpinning the determination of mental disorder depends on whether one considers that the underlying construct is a true category, qualitatively different from other disordered as well as normal states, or whether in fact caseness simply reflects difficulties in functioning at the extreme end of a continuum. Although most psychiatric disorders, child and adult alike, can be shown to be quantitatively different from "normal" states, such differences do not necessarily reflect qualitative differences. Large differences between two groups on a number of markers does not necessarily make them different in kind, any more than tall persons and short persons are from two different species simply because there appears to be a "tall syndrome"—weighing a lot, having long fingers, and wearing big hats. Both quantitative and qualitative distinctions are needed to make an effective argument that a "mental disorder" requires the presence of differences in kind. Finding different kinds *might* constitute a partial argument in support of a particular definition of mental disorder, yet both quantitative and qualitative differences are needed to make the case for different kinds. But two different kinds, even when such can be identified, may have the same final common pathway, in terms of the observable phenomenology, just as two cases of the same kind may have very different outcomes, making the sole use of qualitative distinctions as an indicator of mental disorder problematic (Andreasen et al., 1988). To use the model of height, it is not being short or tall alone that makes someone "patho-

logically" short as opposed to normally short. It may be other associated factors, such as the presence of a disturbance in an endocrine
system or bone metabolism (Eisenberg, 1995).

At present, there is little evidence to indicate *natural* dichotomies
between "cases" and "noncases" in child and adolescent psychopathology. That is, even for disorders for which a great deal of empirical evidence has been brought to bear on the selection of thresholds between normality and disorder in DSM-IV (e.g., Lahey et al.,
1994), DSM-IV diagnoses are perhaps best considered to represent
conventional judgments more than natural dichotomies. This has led
many scholars to advocate *dimensional* approaches to the definition
and assessment of child and adolescent psychopathology rather than
categorical diagnostic approaches. Yet both clinical practice and policy making often require dichotomous decisions about the mental
health of youths. Clinicians must make dichotomous decisions to
treat or withhold treatment on a daily basis; researchers seek to clas-
sify the "phenotypes" of psychopathology to conduct genetic studies;
and policy makers often engage in activities such as counting the
number of youths who need mental health services, but have not received them. Thus, there is a tension between the need for categorical
definitions of mental disorder for many important purposes and the
lack of evidence to support such dichotomous categorizations.

Cutoffs and Their Determination

Because qualitative distinctions have been difficult to demonstrate,
and even when demonstrable, do not appear to be a fully trustworthy
guide to caseness determination, most investigators have relied on
some more or less arbitrary cutoff on a severity or impairment di-
mension to determine caseness. Other than severity and impairment,
other factors that have been considered as potential cutoffs for determination of mental disorder include family members' acknowledg-
ment of the need for treatment, their considering the child's condition
a "problem," and the degree of family burden (Angold et al., 1998).
At least in part, the search for appropriate cutoffs has been spurred
on by the fact that the sole application of DSM criteria has yielded
implausibly high rates of disorder for those wanting to make argu-
ments for parity of health coverage for these conditions (Regier et al.,
1998; Spitzer, 1998). In addition, the presence of a diagnosis does

not necessarily indicate the need for treatment, any more than the presence of a mild upper respiratory infection or warts necessitates commitment of health care dollars or treatment resources—even though most would agree that such conditions are not "normal" from the perspective of actual differences in tissue structure and/or function.

The Impairment Criterion

The most common cutoff applied to determine mental disorder caseness is the construct of impairment, such that in order to present a true case of disorder, one must suffer from some degree of impairment. This is an interesting distinction, and one not necessarily applied equally to other supposed disorders. Hypertension, for many persons, involves no apparent impairment, at least at the present time, and treatment is employed because of the statistical likelihood of future impairment as a result of the untreated condition. In fact, the treatment itself is likely to result in side effects that could be reasonably construed as impairment.

Even accepting the need for impairment, the problem of determining the precise cutoff for the degree of impairment is inescapable. Although a number of strategies have been employed to minimize the numbers of false positives and false negatives (Hsiao et al., 1989; Lahey et al., 1994; Piacentini et al., 1992), such strategies must still rely on some other criterion against which the determination of a "false" positive or negative is made. How much impairment, and as judged by whom? Although the requirement of impairment seems a comfortable position at first glance, close inspection reveals that the many definitions of impairment can yield dramatically different rates of disorder (Angold et al., 1999).

In part, the current requirement for impairment as embodied in the DSM-IV stems from the fact that for mental disorders, children's as well as adults', we have no sure knowledge of the underlying disease processes. Just as with hypertension, the presence of an asymptomatic malignant tumor, although not resulting in current impairment, is known to have certain consequences if left untreated—hence medical necessity is generally taken for granted. From a symptomatic perspective, these might be viewed as analogues to mental disorders' "subthreshold" conditions. For example, once we have obtained reli-

able markers for the likelihood of future onsets of autism or schizophrenia, prevention and early intervention strategies become possible. Eisenberg (1995) has noted that as science progresses, so do our
assumptions of what constitutes mental disorder. More than 100
years ago, knowledge of hemoglobinopathies such as thalassemia
was limited to the overt description of the clinical phenomenology of
symptoms and affected bodily organs. After decades of research,
precise knowledge of the point mutations in the molecular structure
of the hemoglobin molecule underlying these conditions is now available, and persons totally symptomatic can be identified and are considered "cases" from the perspective of prevention, early intervention, and genetic counseling. With time, better knowledge of the
basic neural, psychological, and social processes underlying the mental disorders should allow us to worry less about what should be a
"case" and more about the health merits and ethical issues involved
in intervening with an illness process that is reasonably well understood, at least in terms of prediction of subsequent health impairments.

Global versus Diagnosis-Specific Impairment?

Beyond these initial conceptual difficulties with the requirement of
impairment to establish mental disorder, the measure of impairment,
when actually operationalized and implemented, poses new problems. For example, some instruments that have been developed to assess impairment measure overall impairment (e.g., Piacentini et al.,
1992; Shaffer et al., 1983). Other strategies to measure impairment
attempt to assign the degree of impairment attributable to specific
symptoms or syndromes, such as "diagnosis-specific impairment"
within the Diagnostic Interview Schedule for Children (Shaffer et al.,
1996). Yet when a child has multiple symptoms and/or comorbid
conditions, just how well can one attribute specific aspects of impairment to specific symptoms? Likewise, when one uses a global measure of impairment and employs some cutoff on that measure to
determine which cases appear to meet disorder threshold, the frequently occurring comorbidities would result in some mild cases of
anxiety disorder considered to be above the threshold, simply by virtue of the fact that the particular child had an accompanying severe
conduct disorder. Yet another child with a similar mild anxiety disor-

der would not be determined "a case," simply because he or she had no severe comorbid disorder. Moreover, what if some aspects of the child's impairment are actually attributable to other sources, such as mental retardation? The inability to parse out such aspects of overall impairment in functioning would result in mild instances of disorder being attributed "case" status if accompanied by mental retardation, while similarly mild conditions in children with normal intelligence would not. To our best knowledge, these problems have not received any systematic research attention, nor do we know the impact of such varying methods for determining impairment on prevalence, comorbidity, course of disorder, treatment response, and outcome.

One means of at least partially skirting this problem is instantiated in the Child and Adolescent Psychiatric Assessment (CAPA; Angold & Costello, 2000), where a symptom or criterion is accorded such status only if it is accompanied by impairment. In essence, mild symptoms by definition are not of interest if not accompanied by indicators of distress or disability. This strategy appears promising, but it may also involve a definition sleight of hand: although the definitional approach seems to avoid the problem altogether, it begs the question of whether an interviewer can precisely determine the extent to which a symptom is impairing, especially when it occurs in the context of many other symptoms and adverse life circumstances.

Cultural and Contextual Considerations

As noted by commentators on most recent versions of the DSM, cultural factors play an important role in determining when a "symptom" is a symptom, what constitutes impairment, and cases that need treatment. Rogler (1993) noted that fine-grained analyses of psychotic symptoms with highly structured diagnostic instruments are difficult to make without knowledge of the culture's social values and traditions. Even when question items are appropriately translated, the language and culture may use constructs that do not map neatly onto the DSM. For example, Manson (1995) noted that one item from the Diagnostic Interview Schedule (DIS) that combined guilt, shame, and sinfulness required three different questions among members of the Hopi, in order to avoid confounding different items and meanings. Rogler notes that the configuring of symptoms into disorders may require some changes from culture to culture, yet few studies have taken these issues fully into account. By way of exception, Canino and colleagues (1987), in implementing an epidemiological survey of Puerto Rico, not only conducted tests to ascertain the reliability and validity of the diagnostic instruments, but, as needed, added new items and changed algorithms for various disorders in Puerto Rico. As a consequence of these changes, they found 66% lower disorder rates of obsessive–compulsive disorder than found with the unadjusted diagnostic algorithms. In contrast, dysthymia was 60% higher (Rogler, 1993) when adjusting for cultural factors.

Within a given culture, symptoms, impairment, and mental disorder are likely to be defined in the context of what is expected and "normal" within that culture, rather than on the basis of some underlying etiologic process or biologic substrate (Cantwell, 1996). Given this likelihood, it becomes more apparent that DSM-IV may have set for itself a nearly impossible task, trying to accomplish a reliable description for all possible purposes, even though "purposes" are likely to vary greatly from setting to setting and culture to culture. For example, as derived from various studies of children in Puerto Rico (Piacentini et al., 1992; Shaffer et al., 1996), although parents of Puerto Rican children rate their children as having somewhat more symptoms on the Child Behavior Checklist and similar levels of symptoms on face-to-face diagnostic interviews using the Diagnostic Interview Schedule for Children (as compared with mainland U.S. samples), they attribute much lower levels of overall impairment to those same symptoms than parents of mainland children (Shaffer et al., 1996).

Rather than reifying "mental disorder" as simple symptom counts that cross some relatively arbitrary threshold, Rogler (1993) suggests that within given cultures, a quick decision with substantial face validity can be accomplished for many purposes to avoid attributing symptom, case, or impairment status to conditions or situations that actually reflect some form of goal-directed, culturally situated behavior. Although this is eminently sensible, we are unaware of any systematic testing of such approaches to determine if they can be reliably done, and whether multiple culturally informed raters would agree among themselves with such "face valid" decisions. Although this recommendation hearkens back to the etiological diagnostic formulations of previous DSMs, such an approach, if cautiously implemented, even in Anglo-American cultures, may help avoid according mental disorder status to some conditions that many would regard instead as adaptive responses (e.g., certain forms of conduct disorder; Richters & Cicchetti, 1993) and avoid criticisms that our diagnostic approaches too often ignore the obvious (Jensen & Hoagwood, 1997).

In an important sense, expert clinicians' judgments concerning symptom, impairment, and mental disorder status that make use of all available data over time are an irreplaced "LEAD" (Longitudinal, Expert, and making use of All available Data) (Spitzer, 1983) if not gold standard, yet such judgments too are situated in culture and time, reflecting in part both scientific findings and cultural norms (Eisenberg, 1995). As culture changes or science advances, these determinations do as well. To this extent, the judgment of what constitutes a "case" (in terms of medical necessity or need for treatment) can never be fully satisfied by statistical approaches or complex equations and must instead take into account societal values, willingness to pay, determination of what constitutes a "problem in living" versus a disorder (such as the boundaries between transient sadness and major depressive disorder), as well as the assembled experience and norms of the expert mental health care providers within that cultural context. Without some metric that has carefully calibrated itself by taking into account these dimensions, any determination of "mental disorder" (apart from scientifically established qualitative differences in underlying disease processes) must remain more or less arbitrary.

Children's Caretaking Environments

Important contextual considerations concerning impairment pertain to the finding that under many circumstances, persons may be impaired, yet their symptom pictures are such that they do not fit full DSM criteria. For example, Angold and colleagues (1999) have recently noted that a substantial subset of children evidence quite substantial impairment, yet these children often meet only the criteria for various V codes. Nonetheless, along a number of important external validators, these same children can be shown to suffer substantially and can benefit from treatment. Most frequently, these difficulties are problems concerning their external surroundings, particularly their caretaking environments. Although such difficulties might also be considered "problems in living," a substantial body of evidence suggests that it is just such factors that are related to the onset and persistence of diagnosable conditions. To the extent that such conditions may reflect pathogenic processes that result in the current suffering and may consolidate over time into an enduring pattern of problematic behavior, such situations may be on par with other latent disease processes whose effects are seen only over time (e.g., hypertension), yet which are afforded full mental disorder status. To address this problem, Angold and colleagues recommend that greater use be made of the Not Otherwise Specified (NOS) category, inasmuch as these children usually need and benefit from care at the same levels as those who meet traditional DSM disorder status. Similarly, Emde (1994) and others have suggested that alternative diagnostic schemas are required to include "relationship disorders," particularly in the early years of life. However, such schemas might also be applicable to other ages. But in young children, individual problems are so imbedded in the caregiving relationships that their primary diagnostic location may need to occur at the level of the relationship, because interventions and process-based understanding are most explanatory at that level of analysis (Anders, 1992). There are other approaches to this problem, including the development of new axes (Group for the Advancement of Psychiatry Committee on the Family, 1996), but these ideas at this point have not received widespread acceptance.

Combining Information from Multiple Informants

Unlike most adults who present for clinical care, children are brought in by their parents, usually because of the parents' concerns and wish for assistance, rather than the child's. Under such circumstances, differences in opinions about the nature of the difficulties are common—not just between parent and child, but between parents, or between the parents and the child's teacher. Apart from stipulating the presence of a required set of symptoms with accompanying impairment, sometimes across multiple settings (in the case of attention-deficit/hyperactivity disorder, or ADHD), it is unclear whether the specified number of symptoms must come from a single informant or multiple informants (Cantwell, 1996). A case in point can be seen with the diagnosis of oppositional defiant disorder (ODD). Although this entity was described by clinicians who had seen many parents who presented with children with persistent, severe behavioral difficulties, once operationalized in the DSM, there were no clear guidelines from clinicians to determine *how* "true" cases of disorder should be established, in terms of whether the diagnostic criteria of the disorder should be derived solely from parents, from the child him- or herself, teachers, or even siblings (Cantwell, 1996). Yet once investigators fully explicated the DSM criteria and established companion procedures for obtaining the information from various informants via lay interviewers using structured or semistructured interviews, the researchers' goal of implementing reliable procedures led to obtaining the same information from several informants and, commonly, accepting all positive accounts at face value without any procedures for reconciling discrepancies—very much *unlike* clinical diagnostic procedures. Under such conditions, the likely inclusion of many children as "cases" who would not have met such criteria with the use of standard clinical interviewing procedures seems all too apparent, possibly confounding the clinicians' goal of determining which cases need care with the researchers' goal of implementing replicable procedures with high fidelity.

A number of strategies have been employed to date to address the thorny issues of if, when, and how to combine and/or reconcile discrepant information from different informants. Because most studies have indicated poor symptom and diagnostic agreement between parents and children, many investigators have concluded that parents and children both provide unique, meaningful information that is internally consistent and stable in test–retest studies (Bird et al., 1992; Rubio-Stipec et al., 1994, 1996). As a result, the commonly accepted practice has been to combine information from all informants to generate DSM diagnoses. With the use of such an approach, a child may meet diagnostic criteria based on the parent's report of symptoms, the child's report, or some combination of the two informants' reports—using the "OR" rule (Bird et al., 1992). Although no other algorithms seem to outperform the OR rule in constructing a DSM diagnosis in research settings (Bird et al., 1992), there are many problems inherent in this approach. For example, basing computer-generated diagnoses on the simple OR rule, including the two independent reporters (parent and child), has yielded implausibly high prevalence rates, just as requiring that the symptoms be endorsed by both informants yields excessively low rates (Bird et al., 1992). More important, such an approach does not make clinical sense, because there are often a priori reasons that clinicians would tend to give greater credence to some types of information from certain informants, as compared with other informants.

As one means of addressing this problem, some investigators have recommended that all diagnostic and risk factor information should be considered "informant-specific" (Boyle et al., 1996; Offord et al., 1996). In other words, rather than attempt to reconcile discrepant information, these investigators suggest that researchers treat both sources of data as informative, discarding neither, and using such information to advance knowledge of risk factors and children's outcomes. We agree that this can be a useful empirical strategy, but only for certain purposes. Such a heuristic approach may not give sufficient guidance as to what *should* indicate "mental disorder" for prevalence or policy purposes. Furthermore, this approach may relativize the validity of the information obtained and obscure eventual understanding of valid risk and protective factors. This strategy, if broadly implemented, could lead researchers to spend unnecessary amounts of time trying to understand purported risk factors for a given disorder, when in fact the informant on whom they have relied has provided invalid information. Such research runs the risk of not yielding knowledge of risk factors for a given disorder, but, rather, knowledge of risk factors for a given informant's *perception of disorder.*

Of note, two studies have attempted to address some of these concerns. Interpretation of the first study (Angold & Costello, 1996) is problematic in that it focused solely on ODD, lacked any direct contrasts between parent-only and child-only ODD diagnoses, and did not use any clinical validation procedures. The second study, by Jensen and colleagues (1999), drew upon data from the Methodology for the Epidemiology of Child and Adolescent (MECA) disorders study, examining all cases where parents and children provided discrepant reports of caseness, based on structured diagnostic interviews. Most child-only and parent-only identified (i.e., discrepant) diagnoses were similarly related to impairment and clinical validation, with two exceptions: child-only identified ADHD and ODD. The approach employed in this study appears promising, but requires a different level of conceptual analysis than has been employed for most epidemiologic purposes to date, in order to reconcile differences between various informants. Also of note, other authors have begun to report the use of "discrepancy interviews" as a means of reconciling discrepant information to arrive at the most parsimonious description of the child's actual symptoms, but such procedures have not been rigorously tested and will require additional testing before widespread use (Bidaut-Russell et al., 1995; Nguyen et al., 1994).

The question of "caseness for what purpose" must be considered here as well. Combining informants using an OR rule, coupled with a sufficiently stringent impairment criterion, may work well for addressing practical issues such as who needs care, but the scientific aims of identifying valid syndromes, their risk factors, courses, and outcomes presuppose that a simple perception or report of a symptom or disorder is insufficient, and that when discrepant, various "rules of evidence" (not unlike those a clinician might use to sift through, evaluate, and weigh discrepant information before deciding what the "facts" are) can be employed to some advantage to further the scientific aims of accurate description. Yet as noted earlier, discussion and testing of these strategies within nonclinical settings (e.g., for epidemiologic studies) is in the early stages. Within clinical research settings with instruments such as the Kiddie SADS (Schedule for Affective Disorders and Schizophrenia), resolution of discrepancies is essential, and taken for granted.

Mental Disorder Definitions for Different Ages, Ethnic Groups, or Genders

It is not clear at this point if the most valid definitions of child and adolescent psychopathology should or should not differ according to the age, gender, or ethnicity of the youth. Similarly, we do not now know if different measures of distress and impairment would optimize the identification of impaired cases in youths of different ages, genders, and ethnicities, apart from the cultural factors noted earlier. It is possible that different symptoms, or different symptom thresholds, identify impaired youths at different ages or with different demographic characteristics, but this has not been adequately examined to date. Some evidence in this regard can be found in examining national norms that have been developed for instruments such as the Child Behavior Checklist, where youths of differing ages and genders had differing symptom profiles and actual symptom levels, yet it is not clear how this information should map onto definitions of mental disorder (Achenbach, 1995). Although an array of epidemiological evidence suggests that children of different ages and genders are at a greater risk for various disorders and comorbidities (Nottelmann

& Jensen, 1995), beyond differences in rates, it is not clear whether there are actually different syndromes in these subgroups.

It seems unlikely that we will identify differences in psychopathology related to age, gender, and ethnicity unless we look for them, however. Future studies that allow comparisons between representative samples of youths of different ages, genders, and ethnicities should include diagnostic criteria for which differences might be expected. For example, in the study of gender differences in psychopathology, the inclusion of items describing "relational aggression" (Crick et al., 1997) may reveal gender differences in conduct disorder that would not be identified if these items were not included. In the case of ethnic differences, the inclusion of the few symptoms of *attaque de nervios* that are not included in other DSM-IV syndromes would allow us to determine if this potential culturally specific syndrome is found in Hispanic adolescents, but not in adolescents from other ethnic groups. The inclusion of a small number of such additional items in future population-based studies would be of great importance to the understanding of potential age, gender, and ethnic differences in psychopathology.

In conducting studies that address demographic differences in psychopathology, however, we must be alert for interactions between the demographic characteristics of the youths and the informants. For example, gender differences in youths may be different when the informant on the youth's psychopathology is a female parent or teacher as opposed to a male parent or teacher (Jensen et al., 1988a, 1988b). Similarly, it is possible that the ethnicity of the informant (or the interviewer) and the ethnicity of the youth may interact in the study of ethnic differences in psychopathology. If sample sizes are sufficient, however, it is an easy matter to study and control for such interactions. For epidemiologic studies, this may require strategic oversampling of smaller demographic groups, however.

A final consideration that is important in addressing the question of caseness in children and adolescents is the issue of children's actual trajectories of functioning. Given the rapidly evolving nature of the child's burgeoning capacities, important information can be gleaned from the *rate* of the child's growth and development, and evidence of delays (e.g., failure to thrive, mental or growth retardation) may constitute grounds for consideration of caseness. A major impediment to such issues in the case of children and adolescents is the fact that as currently implemented, diagnostic criteria are static across ages, and as a general rule, symptoms presenting at most ages are taken at face value without consideration of the extent to which a given symptom (e.g., motor activity, inattention, fears of specific objects, separation fears, aggression toward others, etc.) may actually be normative at given ages. Although there is not good evidence to date that such considerations make any difference (e.g., Ryan et al., 1987), these issues have been insufficiently explored, and studies that have examined these questions have been likely greatly underpowered, particularly when examining these issues in nonclinical settings.

SO WHAT DOES THE SENSIBLE CLINICIAN DO? WHAT SHOULD THIS CLINICIAN DO?

In our view, the experienced clinician takes the aforementioned issues into account (i.e., not placing too much emphasis on categorical versus dimensional distinctions, distinguishing diagnosis from the need for treatment, examining the impact of cultural factors on diagnosis and impairment, evaluating the role of context and caretaking factors, evaluating and, when appropriate, combining information from multiple informants, and carefully considering developmental factors). In an attempt to characterize this process, we suggest that a reasonable clinician takes the following steps, though not necessarily in this order:

1. Determine the nature of the presenting problems/chief complaints—determining who needs help and why.
2. Evaluate the developmental nature of symptoms.
3. Examine the cultural and contextual factors affecting presentations.
4. Ascertain levels of impairment.
5. Understand key aspects of the syndrome.
6. Determine the presence of comorbidity and other factors that may affect choice and/or ordering of treatments.

In contrast to research-based approaches that often focus principally on assessing symptoms primarily conceptualized as "within the child," working with these additional considerations requires a life-history approach to diagnosis. "Accurate diagnosis [is] much more akin to detective work or archeology—a quasijudicial procedure,"

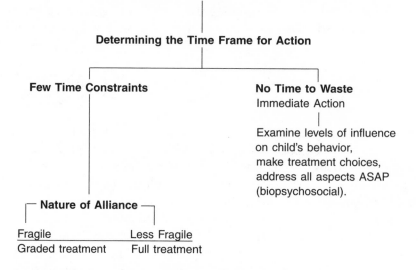

Determination of the Number/Nature of Presenting Problems
(e.g., relative mix of biological, psychological,
and social–environmental factors)

Establishment of Trust:
Formation of a shared view (between therapist and family members)
of the problem, incorporating as feasible the family's beliefs and value systems

Determining the Time Frame for Action

Few Time Constraints

No Time to Waste
Immediate Action

Examine levels of influence
on child's behavior,
make treatment choices,
address all aspects ASAP
(biopsychosocial).

┌─ **Nature of Alliance** ─┐

Fragile
Graded treatment

Less Fragile
Full treatment

Examine levels of influence on child's behavior,
make treatment choices in a graded manner,
based on nature of "resistance" and alliance
(e.g., bio +/– psycho +/– social).

FIGURE 2.1. Clinician's initial treatment decision making: A schematic.

according to Meehl (1973). Schematically we show in Figure 2.1 how a sensible clinician might then approach the complex mass of information presented by a patient and family, and how this clinician organizes his or her approach to intervention. It should be noted that such an approach to intervention does not necessarily presume the same approach or prioritization of etiological factors.

As suggested by Figure 2.1, there exist a number of moderating factors that may affect the clinician's choice or recommendations in the ordering, timing, and/or combining of treatments. Drawing from and expanding the diagram in Figure 2.1, such factors include (1) the child's degree of impairment (with more impairment, most clinicians will increase the range, type, and amount of treatments); (2) interference with developmental lines (with presumed interference, the clinician may be more likely to make/suggest environmental modifications that serve to increase the child's developmental opportunities, with the assumption that normal developmental processes will take hold if not otherwise thwarted); (3) the responsiveness of the problem to intervention type(s) (all things being equal, the clinician is likely to recommend/choose specific treatments known to impact the disorder/symptom/type of impairment); and (4) setting-specificity of the problem and the intervention (if problems are setting-specific, the clinician is likely to target the intervention to that setting).

In addition to these considerations, however, several other principles are likely to operate to guide clinicians' interventions.

Individualized Clinical Approach

Given the enormous complexity of the range of factors shaping a child's clinical presentation, treatment approaches must embed and tailor the intervention within the child's specific developmental stage/status and ecological niche. Such considerations mean that the clinician must of necessity take into careful account whether an intervention will be implemented in a single setting or must cross multiple settings (e.g., home and/or school), whether it should focus on one or multiple domains of functioning (e.g., self-concept, parent–child behavior management, and/or peer relationships), and how it should incorporate the family values and inputs into the treatment design and selection.

Almost no areas of medicine use a "one size fits all" approach to treating pathology: medication dosages are adjusted to body size or surface area, the pace and order of cancer chemotherapies are changed to address individual patients' type and severity of side effects, and even surgical procedures are modified to be better tolerated by frail or compromised patients. Likewise, a good clinician "worth his or her salt" does not continue with a tightly focused didactic approach with parents if significant dissension between parents threatens to scuttle the entire therapeutic enterprise. Nor does a skilled therapist continue trying to "unload" his or her therapeutic goods on a family if overarching issues of trust/distrust or like/dislike seem to be undermining the family's confidence in the therapist's abilities. Yet too many modern-day managed-care-driven treatments seem to forget that these issues are paramount to the integrity of the treatment.

Parents and Families as Partners in the Therapeutic Process

To address concerns about the palatability of our therapies to families, an effective clinician is usually very attentive to the relationship to children and families as *partners* in the therapeutic process. Therapies that fail to build this principle into the approach to families are likely to miss a critical component of treatment effectiveness. Unlike more traditional biomedical procedures that are presumably active once the intervention has been delivered or ingested (e.g., medications), the psychotherapies are inextricably intertwined with the psychopathologic conditions to the extent that both are embedded in behavioral patterns of human social exchange. Without the full enlistment of all critical family members in using their behaviors to change the child's behaviors, success is much less certain. This recruitment of family effort is possible only to the extent that the therapy itself represents a *partnership* between therapist and family participants, and to the degree that the therapist communicates this principle effectively and convincingly to these would-be therapeutic partners. Such partnerships, both in the course of pharmaco- and/or psychotherapy, are key to long-term success.

Putting It All Together: Understanding and Applying Principles of Behavior Change

Clinicians should proceed with treatment only if (1) they possess a clear theory and/or understanding of the principles of treatment (e.g., what are the *necessary though not sufficient* elements of change in this treatment paradigm?); (2) given these therapeutic principles, they know what types of person- or family-specific obstacles may hamper the delivery and effectiveness of the treatment (including the family's commitment to the *therapeutic partnership*); and (3) they know which modifications in pace, ordering, and timing of treatments must be accommodated in order to minimize the effects of these potential obstacles on the active components of treatment. For example, an overarching hierarchy of therapeutic principles (based on the clinician's best "wisdom") might be constructed that supersede (or must precede) the implementation of an effective psychosocial intervention. Such principles might include the family's/parents' need for control/autonomy in directing family affairs, the apparent consistency of an intervention with the family's values, sufficient marital harmony so that both parents can actively support the intervention, trust and/or liking for the therapist, the apparent sensibility/credibility of the intervention to the family, the "fairness" of the intervention to family members affected by it, the family partners' ability to "attend to" and learn the intervention, and the presence of appropriate/sufficient emotional reserves and equilibrium in those who must deliver and receive the intervention.

The presence of these factors, coupled with elements/principles of change, may together constitute the *necessary* and *sufficient* ingredients to deliver a reasonably effective psychosocial intervention with an active treatment component. Yet in a *therapeutic partnership*, it is likely that some autonomy must be surrendered to the partner/therapist (if change is to occur), but this best occurs in the presence of trust, liking, and confidence in the therapist. If the intervention is inconsistent with family members' values, seems unfair, or "just doesn't make sense" from their perspective, it will take a very high degree of trust before such an intervention can proceed (if at all), or else the differences in therapist and family values and treatment rationale must be fully adjudicated. Likewise, the presence of marital difficulties, preoccupation with other problems, or severe emotional distress (sadness, anger, anxiety) in any of the therapeutic partners must be monitored. Just as the cancer chemotherapist delays the delivery of more antitumor agents when the platelet count drops too low, the psychotherapist monitors these core emotional levels within the family therapeutic partners, and at critical junctures addresses these issues directly, all in the service of providing the most effective psychotherapy for the child's identified difficulties.

We close this chapter by noting the enormity of the assessment challenges that face a clinician who attempts to deal with a troubled child and concerned family. Diagnoses not only fall short, but they also often fail to capture the critical issues of context, development, and the nature of the child's fit within his or her particular setting. Yet it is difficult for the clinician to keep so many issues and clinical principles in view when facing this assessment challenge. We suggest that there are indeed models that are simultaneously developmental, contextual, and adaptational, and that accord with much of the basic research that guides modern-day biology. These approaches, which rely on biological systems theory can take into account evolutionary theory for understanding symptoms and disorders. We find these considerations quite "sympatico" with much of our work as clinicians. The following chapter discusses some of the basic issues in evolutionary and adaptational theory, and then, because this perspective illuminates how clinicians often approach children during the evaluation and treatment processes, subsequent chapters apply this approach to specific disorders and syndromes.

REFERENCES

Achenbach TM (1995) Empirically based assessment and taxonomy: Applications to clinical research. *Psychol Assess*, 7:261–274.

Anders TF (1992) Clinical syndromes, relationship disturbances, and their assessment. In AJ Sameroff & RN Emde (Eds.), *Relationship disturbances in early childhood: A developmental approach* (pp. 125–144). New York: Basic Books.

Andreasen NC, Shore D, Burke JD, Grove WM, et al. (1988) Clinical phenomenology. *Schizoph Bull*, 14:345–363.

Angold A & Costello EJ (1996) The relative diagnostic utility of child and parent reports of oppositional defiant behaviors. *In J Methods Psychiatr Res*, 6:253–259.

Angold A & Costello EJ (2000) The Child and Adolescent Psychiatric Assessment (CAPA). *J Am Acad Child Adolesc Psychiatry*, 39:39–48.

Angold A, Costello EJ, Farmer EM, Burns BJ, & Erkanli A (1999) Impaired but undiagnosed. *J Am Acad Child Adolesc Psychiatry*, 38:129–137.

Angold A, Messer SC, Stangl D, et al. (1998) Perceived parental burden and service use for child and adolescent psychiatric disorders. *Am J Public Health*, 88:75–80.

Bidaut-Russell M, Reich W, Cottler LB, et al, (1995) The Diagnostic Interview Schedule for Children (PC-DISC v 3.0): Parents and adolescents suggest reasons for expecting discrepant answers. *J Abnorm Child Psychol*, 23:641–659.

Bird HR, Gould MS, & Staghezza B (1992) Aggregating data from multiple informants in child psychiatry epidemiological research. *J Am Acad Child Adolesc Psychiatry*, 31:78–85.

Boyle MH, Offord DR, Racine Y, Szatmari P, Fleming JE, & Sanford M (1996) Identifying thresholds for classifying childhood psychiatric disorder: Issues and prospects. *J Am Acad Child Adolesc Psychiatry*, 35:1440–1448.

Canino GJ, Bird HR, Shrout PE, et al. (1987). The prevalence of specific psychiatric disorders in Puerto Rico. *Arch Gen Psychiatry*, 44:727–735.

Cantwell DP (1996) Classification of child and adolescent psychopathology. *J Child Psychol Psychiatry Allied Disciplines*, 37:3–12.

Crick NR, Casa JF, & Mosher M (1997) Relational and overt aggression in preschool. *Developmental Psychol*, 33:579–588.

Eisenberg L (1995) *Doing away with the illusion of homogeneity: Medical progress through disease identification*. First Leo Kanner Lecture, Division of Child and Adolescent Psychiatry, Johns Hopkins Hospital, Baltimore.

Emde R (1994) Individuality, context, and the search for meaning. *Child Dev*, 65:719–737.

Frances A (1998) Problems in defining clinical significance in epidemiological studies. *Arch Gen Psychiatry*, 55:119.

Group for the Advancement of Psychiatry Committee on the Family (1996) Global Assessment of Relational Functioning scale (GARF): I. Background and rational. *Fam Process*, 35:155–172.

Hsiao JK, Bartko JJ, & Potter WZ (1989) Diagnosing diagnoses: Receiver operating characteristic methods and psychiatry. *Arch Gen Psychiatry*. 46:664–667.

Jensen PS & Hoagwood K (1997) The book of names: DSM-IV in context. *Dev Psychopathology*, 9:231–249.

Jensen PS & Members of the MTA Cooperative Group (2002) ADHD comorbidity findings from the MTA study: New diagnostic subtypes and their optimal treatments. In JE Helzer & JJ Hudziak (Eds.), *Defining psychopathology in the 21st century: DSM-V and beyond* (pp. 169–192). Washington, DC: American Psychiatric Publishing.

Jensen PS, Rubio-Stipec M, Canino G, Bird HR, Dulcan MK, Schwab-Stone ME, & Lahey BB (1999) Parent and child contributions to diagnosis of mental disorder: Are both informants always necessary? *J Am Acad Child Adolesc Psychiatry*, 38:1569–1579.

Jensen PS, Traylor J, Xenakis SN, & Davis H (1988a) Child psychopathology rating scales and interrater agreement: I. Parents' gender and psychiatric symptoms. *J Am Acad Child Adolesc Psychiatry*, 27:442–450.

Jensen PS, Xenakis SN, Davis H, & Degroot J (1988b) Child psychopathology rating scales and interrater agreement: II. Child and family characteristics. *J Am Acad Child Adolesc Psychiatry*, 27:451–461.

Kendler KS & Gardner CO (1998) Boundaries of major depression: An evaluation of DSM-IV criteria. *Am J of Psychiatry*, 155:172–177.

Kirk SA & Hsieh DK (2004) Diagnostic consistency in assessing conduct disorder: An experiment on the effect of social context. *Am J Orthopsychiatry*, 74:43–55.

Lahey BB, Applegate B, McBurnett K, Biederman J, Greenhill L, Hynd GW, Barkley RA, Newcorn J, Jensen P, Richters J, et al. (1994) DSM-IV trials for attention deficit hyperactivity disorder in children and adolescents. *Am J of Psychiatry*, 151:1673–1685.

Levy F, Hay DA, McStephen M, Wood C, & Waldman I (1997) Attention-deficit hyperactivity disorder: A category or continuum? Genetic analysis of a large-scale twin study. *J Am Acad Child Adolesc Psychiatry*, 36:737–744.

Manson SM (1995) Culture and major depression: Current challenges in the diagnosis of mood disorders. *Psychiatr Clin North Am*. 18:487–501.

Meehl PE (1973) When shall we use our heads instead of the formula? In PE Meehl, *Psychodiagnosis: Selected papers* (pp. 81–89). New York: Norton.

Nelson CA & Bloom FE (1997) Child development and neuroscience. *Child Dev*, 68:970–987.

Nguyen N, Whittlesey S, Scimeca K, DiGiacomo D, et al. (1994) Parent–child agreement in prepubertal depression: Findings with a modified assessment method. *J Am Acad Child Adolesc Psychiatry*, 33:1275–1283.

Nottlemann ED & Jensen PS (1995) Bipolar affective disorder in children and adolescents. *J Am Acad Child Adolesc Psychiatry*, 34:705–708.

Offord DR, Boyle MH, Racine Y, Szatmari P, Fleming JE, Sanford M, & Lipman EL (1996) Integrating assessment data from multiple informants. *J Am Acad Child Adolesc Psychiatry*, 35:1078–1085.

Piacentini JC, Cohen P, & Cohen J (1992) Combining discrepant diagnostic information from multiple sources: Are complex algorithms better than simple ones? *J Abnorm Child Psychol*, 20:51–63.

Rasmussen ER, Neuman RJ, Heath AC, Levy F, Hay DA, & Todd RD (2002) Replication of the latent class structure of attention-deficit/hyperactivity disorder (ADHD) subtypes in a sample of Australian twins. *J Child Psychol Psychiatry*, 43:1018–1028.

Regier DA, Rae DS, Narrow WE, Kaelber CT, & Schatzberg AF (1998) Limitations of diagnostic criteria and assessment instruments for mental disorders: Implications for research and policy. *Arch Gen Psychiatry*, 55:109–115.

Richters JE & Cicchetti D (1993) Mark Twain meets DSM-III-R: Conduct disorder, development, and the concept of harmful dysfunction. *Dev Psychopathology*, 5:5–29.

Robins E & Guze SB (1970) Establishment of diagnostic validity in psychiatric illness: Its application to schizophrenia. *Am J Psychiatry*, 126:983–987.

Rogler LH (1993) Culture in psychiatric diagnosis: An issue of scientific accuracy. *Psychiatry*, 56:324–327.

Rubio-Stipec M, Canino GJ, Shrout P, Dulcan M, Freeman D, & Bravo M (1994) Psychometric properties of parents and children as informants in child psychiatry epidemiology with the Spanish Diagnostic Interview Schedule for Children (DISC.2). *J Abnorm Child Psychol*, 122:703–720.

Rubio-Stipec M, Shrout PE, Canino G, Bird HR, Jensen P, Dulcan M, &

Schwab-Stone M (1996) Empirically defined symptom scales using the DISC 2.3. *J Abnorm Child Psychol*, 24:67–83.

Ryan ND, Puig-Antich J, Ambrosini P, Rabinovich H, et al. (1987) The clinical picture of major depression in children and adolescents. *Arch Gen Psychiatry*, 44:854–861.

Shaffer D, Fisher P, Dulcan MK, Davies M, Piacentini J, Schwab-Stone ME, Lahey BB, Bourdon K, Jensen PS, Bird HR, Canino G, & Regier DA (1996) The NIMH Diagnostic Interview Schedule for Children Version 2.3 (DISC-2.3): Description, acceptability, prevalence rates, and performance in the MECA study (Methods for the Epidemiology of Child and Adolescent Mental Disorders Study). *J Am Acad Child Adolesc Psychiatry*, 35:856–877.

Sonuga-Barke EJ (1998) Categorical models of childhood disorder: A conceptual and empirical analysis. *J Child Psychol Psychiatry Allied Disciplines*, 39:115–133.

Spitzer RL (1983) Psychiatric diagnosis: Are clinicians still necessary? *Compr Psychiatry*, 24:399–411.

Spitzer RL (1998) Diagnosis and need for treatment are not the same. *Arch Gen Psychiatry*, 55:119.

Wakefield JC (1992) The concept of mental disorder: On the boundary between biological facts and social values. *Am Psychol*, 47:373–388.

Wakefield JC, Pottick KJ, & Kirk SA (2002). Should the DSM-IV diagnostic criteria for conduct disorder consider social context? *Am J Psychiatry*, 159:380–386.

Wallace ER (1994) Psychiatry and its nosology: A historico-philosophical overview. In JZ Sadler, OP Wiggins, et al. (Eds), *Philosophical perspectives on psychiatric diagnostic classification* (pp. 16–86). Baltimore: Johns Hopkins University Press.

Werry JS, Reeves JC, & Elkind GS (1987) Attention deficit, conduct, oppositional, and anxiety disorders in children: I. A review of research on differentiating characteristics. *J Am Acad Child Adolesc Psychiatry*, 26:133–143.

Zarin DA & Earls F (1993) Diagnostic decision making in psychiatry. *Am J of Psychiatry*, 50:197–206.

CHAPTER 3

Understanding Early Development and Temperament from the Vantage Point of Evolutionary Theory

PENNY KNAPP

EARLY NEURODEVELOPMENTAL EVENTS

The newborn (hereafter, for simplicty, "he") reacts with global excitation or withdrawal to touch, sound, smell, taste, fullness, emptiness, and to the new apparitions in the light outside the womb. Two-thirds of his metabolic energy is dedicated to his brain, which is developing neurons and dendrites, elaborating connections among them (Allman, 1998, p. 175), and furnishing them with glial tissue. He is richly equipped with reflexes and perceptual capacities attuned to respond to the care of a parent (hereafter, for simplicity, "she") (e.g., Eibl-Eibesfeldt, 1989). He would die quickly without it.

Genes

The human genome, redundant and flexible, has resources for adaptive creativity, allowing procreativity. Despite a wide adaptive capacity and a long lifespan, we cannot develop as humans without protracted dependency in infancy. A single mutation may determine a complex behavior pattern (Tuszynski, 1998), but more often, we cannot detect how any one gene is instrumental in the orchestrated development of the adapting organism. During gestation and infancy, hundreds of genes determine or regulate expression of enzymes and biosynthetic pathways in the growth and differentiation of the nervous system (Berretta et al., 1992; Schore, 1997). The activities of these genes, and their expression, are optimized (Hubel & Wiesel, 1979), canalized (Waddington, 1966), or interfered with (Snyder, 1998) by experience, and are responsive to the environment (Morell, 1999). Experience, for a social animal, includes the actions and reactions of other animals.

The newborn brain, an infant survival unit, has evolved to adapt and is equipped to adapt. Adaptation demands negotiating both homeostasis and invention. Self-constructing, each brain negotiates uniquely to adapt to the environment in which it must survive. For the 12 billion-odd human neurons, the minimal environmental need includes interpersonal stimulation (Aitken & Trevarthen, 1997; Emde et al., 1965). The human newborn, helpless to survive alone, is richly equipped to respond to interpersonal cues. In an impoverished environment, development of a young brain is meager (Greenough et al., 1987; Kolb et al., 1998): synapses do not increase, dendrites sprout less, and (Gage et al., 1995) stem cells, which are in continuous production, preferentially differentiate into astroglia rather than neurons.

Advancing development constructs and reconstructs larger and larger cell assemblies and links them together with increasing self-organization. The infant's physiological patterns of regulation and response are mapped. The corticotropin-releasing factor in the paraventricular hypothalamus (Schore, 1997) installs the first settings for a homeostatic stress response system that will operate until death. The functional range of this first homeostatic system will determine the adaptive range and neuronal architecture of the developing brain (Sapolsky, 1992), with potential salutary or adverse consequences (see, e.g., discussion by Sapolsky, 2004).

Experience

To successfully adapt, it is necessary to find a balance between buffering stress and optimizing experience. Stress response systems, as well as seeking and digesting food, are among the oldest developmental organizations. The hypothalamic–pituitary–adrenal (HPA) axis is situated to respond to and regulate stress. Corticotropin-releasing factor (CRF) and/or arginine-vasopressin (AVP) are elicited in the hypothalamus and, together with cholinergic and serotonergic systems, act on the pituitary to release adrenocorticotropic hormone (ACTH). In a positive feedback loop, receptors in the brain are stimulated, action that is mediated through many neurotransmitters. This is the allostatic system, the emergency response system that allows the animal to protect itself from danger.

Understimulation of an infant animal results in less neuronal tissue (Greenough et al., 1987) through blocking of catecholeamine-generated mitochondrial energizing of neuronal growth. Because the infant has not yet developed compensatory mechanisms to buffer prolonged sympathomimetic activity, overstimulation of this allostatic system evokes intense distress. Increased cortisol production is followed by parasympathetic vagal-associated dissociation, with hypoarousal (Perry et al., 1995; Porges, 1995; Porges et al., 1994). Indeed, enough overstimulation of the system, even in the stable and mature individual, produces the same effects, which are termed overarousal and dissociation, respectively. If he is allowed to suffer enduring states of negative painful arousal, the resulting prolonged elevation of the infant's corticosteroid levels alters the metabolic climate in which his brain develops (Schore, 1997; Sapolsky, 2000). Nucleic acid synthesis is curtailed, corticosteroid receptors are decreased, brain energy metabolism is reduced (Bryan, 1990), and dendritic branching is not optimized. Excitatory neurotransmitters may become toxic (Novelli et al., 1988), leading to alteration of mitochondrial structure and function (Kimberg et al., 1968).

Lifelong levels of reactivity of the allostatic system may be established prenatally (e.g., Schneider et al., 1999) and by early experience (Spinelli, 1987), and severe experiences may manifest in permanent resets in noradrenaline levels (Higley et al., 1991; Perry et al., 1995). It is known that intense or repeated stress, either prenatally (Weinstock, 1996) or later in life (Jacobsen & Sapolsky, 1991; Sapolsky et al., 1986) causes excitotoxic apoptosis of receptors, dysregulation of the homeostatic mechanism, and possibly irreversible changes (Kaufer et al., 1999; Sapolsky, 1992). Young animals subjected to excessive stress forfeit some capacity to learn; this has been shown to be mediated through change in number or affinity of receptors in the hypothalamus, the hippocampus, and the amygdala. Experimental manipulations of stress in infant animals delineate the adaptive limits of a delicate and complex system under extreme conditions.

It is a mother's job to stimulate her infant while keeping his stress in a bearable range. Responsivity between mother and infant is immediate, vital, and mutually contingent: face-to-face (Beebe & Lachman, 1988), skin to skin, within each other's voice and aroma. The mother's embracing attentions buffer the infant against the stresses of the environment, as well as those of his own hungers, balancing protection and stimulation. In response, the infant's plasma noradrenaline rises to a catalytic optimum, activating his sympatheic nervous system, increasing brain mitochondrial cytochrome oxidase-rich zones (Purves & LaMantia, 1990), oxygen consumption, and energy metabolism. This catecholamine-generated arousal increases cerebral oxidative energy metabolism from the low newborn level to a cerebral metabolic rate that consumes more than half of total body oxygen consumption during infancy (Allman, 1998, p. 175). This nourishes the proliferation of neurons and dendritic spines and the connections of modular circuits between them.

In the ecological niche of his mother's lap, breast, hands, and voice, the individual's lifetime neurobiological resilience will be the product of this neuronal construction, cast in a balance or imbalance between too much stimulation and not enough.

Homeostasis

Primitive circuits, parallel to the more recently evolved ones, infuse events around and between us with intense emotion, and neuronal links to the allostatic system regulating the stress response remain active. Central to these circuits are the hypothalamus, the hippocampus, and the amygdala. Initially, the response of these circuits is relatively unmodulated.

The newborn's hunger is stormy, his satiation pacific. Aroused by cold or pain, he fills his lungs and flails his limbs with such extremity of sympathetic discharge that he would collapse if he did not switch to a parasympathetic conservation pattern (Porges et al., 1994). Adaptation to a complex world is impossible without enlarging the homeostatic response to stress. This is the project that occupies his mother's days and nights in feeding, bringing up the gassy bubbles, cleaning, cooing, and soothing.

The earliest developing brain systems immediately begin to diversify. Initially, the dynamics of their response have a nonlinear pattern. Rapidly responding primitive brain systems, not yet extensively connected to modulating circuits in the cortex, galvanize the animal. The stochastic pattern of this response is nonlinear and chaotic, so that small perturbations inside the organism may either move the organism toward greater stabilization or initiate logarithmic trajectories to a very different state (Goerner, 1995; Schore, 1997). From an evolutionary point of view, this pattern gives the organism flexibility for adaptation. It may be either a trump card (e.g., if it allows crucial one-trial learning to avoid danger) or a time bomb (e.g., if an experience is traumatic and forecloses compensatory learning).

Later in development, the brain is capable of moderating responses and the individual is able to control the rate and degree of response to situations. Glucocorticoids regulate metabolism and physiological functions in the hippocampus; high doses affect verbal declarative memory but not attention, spatial recognition, or spatial recall (Newcomer et al., 1999). This reversible effect may indicate a trade-off of slower analytic functions for quicker emergency response functions in circumstances of stress (Arnstein, 1999).

Attachment between the mother and infant, and between adults, moderates stress and thus increases resilience. Endocrine systems, inseparable from neurological systems, also serve these behavior patterns well. The central nervous system develops with sexual dimorphism (Gorski, 1999). During fetal development there are gender differences in the number of neurons and their volumes in various nuclei, in synaptic connections between brain regions, and in the regional patterns of expression of various neurochemicals. These differences arise from relative gradients in hormonal concentrations and ratios, rather than from the presence or absence of a specific male or female hormone. The exact time course and functional significance of these dimorphisms are still not known, but links to gender differences in emotional pattern and in cognitive functioning may be proposed. Aggressive initiatives are moderated by androgens, and risk-averse behaviors moderated by estrogen and its actions on serotonin metabolism. Oxytocin and arginine-vasopressin (AVP), venerable hormones that regulate reproduction, are present in both females and males, but their distribution in male species is variable (Insel et al., 1995). Males in monogamous, pair-living species, which also assist in care of their young, have higher oxytocin and AVP levels (Insel & Hulihan, 1995). Gender differences in response to stress may be related to this.

EMOTIONAL RELATEDNESS

The sequence of neuronal proliferation (Aitken & Trevarthen, 1997; Berretta et al., 1992; Schore, 1997; Waddington, 1966) appears to have evolved to select for a capacity for intense interpersonal attachment; this is salvation for a hairless, clawless creature, whose large brain requires it to traverse its mother's pelvis many months before it can survive alone. In the first year and a half of life, the structure of the right hemisphere is cast (Kinney et al., 1988), specifically those biogenic aminergic systems that regulate the activity and growth of the limbic system and right frontotemporal cortical connections to deeper areas. This happens in an experience-dependent fashion (Hubel & Wiesel, 1979; Mishkin & Appenzeller, 1987). The infant's core experiences occur within his attachment to a mothering caregiver. The development that we *see* begin at the breast has actually begun with the notochord in the gastrula and can be supported or jeopardized by that caregiver's care of her own body and her womb within it. It continues through months of nursing and social nurturance. We see the nursing mother and her baby, the teaching mother and her talking toddler; what is happening between them, and how does it affect the young developing brain?

The vital contingent responsivity between mother and infant has been described best with respect to their visual reciprocity (Beebe & Lachman, 1988). This has perhaps occurred because the tools of photograph and video offer themselves so well for this. However, mother and infant are not only face-to-face, but are also skin to skin and close within each other's smell and hearing. The infant is elaborating thousands of neurons and dendrites a day. His physiological patterns of regulation and response are mapped.

All the contingent and noncontingent actions of his caregiver(s) are experiences for the infant. His brain, in a growth boom, lays down neuronal and dendritic connections from these experiences, spending neuronal materials judiciously (Cherniak, 1995), embedding many subsystems within cortical maps (Krubitzer, 1995), and deploying neurotransmitters flexibly. Selective expression of his genes, catalysts of his new learning, and the building, remodeling, and organization of his brain, are modulated by his affective states.

Though utterly dependent, the human baby is far from passive (Calkins et al., 1996; Fox et al., 1994; Schore, 1997). Attachment with the caregiver is active and reciprocal, even as it catalyzes and modulates the infant's experience and thereby influences the architecture and activity of the infant's brain. Winnicott (1990) coined the expression "good-enough mother" to describe the innumerable acts and emotions of a mother who nurtures a thriving infant. The "good-enough mother" is suffused with hormones and neuropeptides; she lactates, lets down her milk, and modulates her own affective states in anticipation of and in response to those of the infant. This relationship builds the baby's neuronal system to express the self-writing software within his brain that programs him for the personal passions and responses that we call his humanity or his symptomatology, depending on our philosophical frame.

Regulation

The early developing brain systems modulate behavior and experience immaturely, and in an unstable fashion. Swings between extremes have been described as demonstrating nonlinear dynamics. This instability predisposes to chaotic responses, so that small perturbations inside the organism may either move the organism toward greater stabilization or initiate logarithmic trajectories to a very different state (Goerner, 1995; Schore, 1997). From an evolutionary point of view, this gives the organism flexibility for adaptation.

The infant's dependence on the caregiver places him at the mercy of the caregiver's ability to buffer stress (Coplan et al., 1996). Titrating the infant's level of excitement to balance tropism against excitotoxic, apoptotic cell death, requires a safe and emotionally stable environment. Transient alterations in noradrenaline levels may become permanent resets (Higley et al., 1991; Perry et al., 1995). If, in the context of attachment, early brain organization proceeds well, there is a balance between excitatory and inhibitory patterns and the developing child has a chance for self regulation within later relationships.

The early developmental experience has cast the pattern of a lifelong need for affiliation, a balance between vulnerability (Wang &

Pitts, 1994) and resiliency (Werner, 1995), a pattern of gratifying intimacy or of fearful maneuvering with others, or infinite permutations between these. Periods of sustained interactive failure, and negative affect between infant and caregiver, result in negative development, because the infant, even in the earliest months of life, has self-directed regulatory behaviors to control negative affect, and these may begin to be triggered indiscriminately and inflexibly (Lieberman & Van Horn, 1998). Around the end of the first year of life, infants develop awareness of their own states and intentions, and of those of their caregivers. This is termed "intersubjectivity" by Tronick (1989), "secondary intersubjectivity" by Trevarthen (Aitken & Trevarthen, 1997), and "attunement" by Stern (1977).

Emotional self-regulation develops iteratively as experience modifies physiology and neurophysiology predisposes response to experience. The concept of temperament, which predisposes stable characteristics of response, is a conceptual summary of the trend for a child. It abstracts multiple observations of how, within the child's nervous system, a balance is being constructed between either postive or negative affects, either inhibited or uninhibited emotional expression, and a pattern of behavioral activation that tends either to approach or to avoid new experiences. The balance may partially reside within the two hemispheres. Relative right frontal hypoactivation in toddlers is associated with aggression (Fox, 1991), anger-proneness, and approach tendencies (Davidson & Fox, 1988; Dawson, 1994).

Parents generate an emotional climate, which has been shown to powerfully influence children's adjustment (Block et al., 1981; McHale & Rasmussen, 1998; Minuchin, 1985). As "cells that fire together, wire together," experience becomes memory, which organizes new experience. Toddlers are capable of deferred imitation of complex action sequences, even after weeks have passed; the interval over which they can remember events increases with age, (Hudson & Sheffield, 1998) and after reenactment, the reinstated memories of early events tend to persist.

Penetrating these developmental trends, and expressed through them, are genetic factors. Certain genetic patterns may have such a powerful effect that the child's earliest experiences barely mitigate them. Others explain but a fraction of the variance in children's development. Moreover, penetrance or expression of genes may vary. Particular clinical outcomes driven by genetic unfolding may be isomorphic with those arising from experience. For example, social withdrawal may be determined by a biological factor with measurable markers (e.g., mitochondrial abnormalities in Rett syndrome) or may be the result of adaptive response to neglect, as in anaclitic depression (Spitz, 1945).

Malleability in the developing child is not unlimited. From the time of their birth, individuals show individuality in the intensity or the sensitivity of their responses. The concept of temperament seeks to describe or dimensionalize this. Polarities such as extraversion versus intraversion, shyness versus aggression, and the "easy" child versus the "difficult" child are examples. Some groups have also included hypersensitivity and hyposensitivity to sensory stimuli within the concept of temperament (e.g., Kagan, 2003), as well as the achievement or nonachievement of regularity in sleeping, eating, and other biological functions in early childhood. These concepts, although descriptively derived, are robust and are found in most cultures. They may approximate neuroregulatory factors predictive of behavioral expression and emotional regulation that might serve as the foundation of a future diagnostic system. Current examples of such research include links to later brainstem auditory evoked response (Woodward et al., 2001) and links to vagal tone (Beauchaine, 2001).

Social Communication

As noted, survival of a social animal requires sensitivity to signals from others and the capacity to send comprehensible signals. Recent findings about inborn behavioral propensities for social interaction suggest that children may be "primed" for social communication. The beginnings of cognitive and social development occur before birth (Karmiloff-Smith, 1995; Locke, 1993). The auditory and visual capacities of newborns can be evaluated using habituation and preferential looking/listening paradigms. Sounds that are repeatedly experienced before birth (especially the mother's voice) become familiar to the baby before birth, and he will selectively orient to them in the first hours after birth (Ockleford et al., 1988). Mehler and his colleagues (Bertoncini et al., 1989) report that at 4 days of age, babies born in France of French-speaking mothers prefer the sound of French to Russian, but babies born in France whose mothers spoke a different language than French lack this preference; indeed, they give little evidence they discriminate either language. Current research suggests that children's learning of language is so rapid as to suggest that innate facilitating mechanisms may play a role. Between 1 and 4 months of age infants learn to distinguish each of the 150 speech sounds that make up all human languages (Kuhl, 1991). By 6 months of age, infants are able to distinguish subtle variants in phonetic characteristics between their native language and other languages (Kuhl et al., 2000).

Newborns emit recognizable facial expressions (interest, joy, surprise, distress) that are appropriate to the nature of events and to their context (Izard, 1994; Malatesta & Izard, 1984; Tronick, 1989). They can also imitate the repeated presentation of certain adult facial movements, including tongue protrusion (Field et al., 1983; Meltzoff & Moore, 1977). Neonates preferentially track a face-like stimulus (three high-contrast blobs in the locations of the eyes and the mouth) in preference to other interesting stimuli (Vecera & Johnson, 1995). By 3 months of age infants frequently display full-face and partial expression of interest, joy, sadness, and anger, and the patterns of muscle movements involved in these expressions remain stable through the first 9 months (Izard, 1994).

Infants actively engage in behaviors that lead directly to better social engagement (e.g., Tronick, 1989). An infant may selectively signal his caretaker that he is ready to interact by looking at her and smiling. Dyadic interaction catalyzes this signaling, to the mutual delight of the pair; mothering persons in all cultures play with infants by initiating routines with enhanced tone of voice, wider facial expression, and exaggerated gestures and body language, a communication pattern called "motherese." Young children readily respond with their own prosodic, facial, and gestural displays. These caregiver–baby sequences, designed to highlight and encourage the types of social signaling that will be important in later social communication, are universal experiences in well-adapted dyads, surpassing those in experimental learning laboratories in persistence and ingenuity. The older infant actively sustains and perpetuates these sequences. If, in an experimental paradigm, a mother is instructed to suddenly stop interacting, a young child will characteristically perceive that something is different and may become upset or look puzzled. The infant may use additional behaviors to control his distress in this situation: looking away, self-comforting, or even self-stimulation. By 12–14 months of age children will respond to others in distress, using empathic patting and facial expressions of concern (Zahn-Wexler et al., 1992).

Similar behavioral propensities are observed in other primates, suggesting evolutionary selection for social behavior. Darwin commented on this in 1873 (e.g., Plutchik, 1980), observing that both humans and other higher primates expressed emotion through the use of facial expression and body posture. Some human gestures and expressions are quite similar to those of other closely related primates, some are not. Darwin's statements were based on anecdotal evidence, but more recent field work has confirmed his beliefs. Chimpanzees show elaborate emotional signaling systems employing facial expression, gesture, and cries (e.g., Brothers, 1989). Like human infants, chimp babies come into the world with the innate capacity to display facial expression of emotions. The innate nature of this phenomenon is shown by the observation that rhesus monkeys reared from birth in complete isolation showed appropriate responses to motion-picture- and slide-presented faces of monkeys displaying fear and threat (Sackett, 1966). Evolutionary survival has apparently selected for human infants to be born prepared to recognize their parents and discern social signals from background noise, and to quickly learn to emit and respond to nonverbal social signals with increasing sophistication and effectiveness.

THE DEVELOPMENT OF JOINT ATTENTION AND THEORY OF MIND

Building on the capacity to emit and respond to social signals and shared emotions, infants soon begin to engage in a higher form of interaction called *joint attention*. This concept encompasses reciprocal babbling, spontaneously sharing food and toys, and attunement of expression and emotional responses. It includes referential communication, in which the child shows interesting objects to his parents or points to interesting objects, looking first at the parent and then at the object, as if to say, "Let's share this." Joint attention actions may serve to direct the attention of an adult to an object and to simultaneously create and enrich a social-emotional encounter.

Scaife and Bruner (1975) provided an early report on the development of joint attention. They reported on the infant's ability to follow another person's signals in attending to a directed observation.

The infant sat in the lap of the investigator, who, after ascertaining that the child was settled and alert, made eye contact with the child, then silently turned her head away to fixate a signal light 1.5 m distant. At 2–4 months of age, only 30% of infants also looked to the light, but by 11–14 months of age 100% of infants did. Older infants may also look back to the investigator after looking toward the light. Other investigators have reported similar findings (e.g., Karmiloff-Smith, 1995).

Beyond 6 months of age children engage in many acts of sharing with their caretakers, and for the first time they show evidence of having what has been called a "theory of mind." When very young children begin to understand that others have minds that differ from theirs, and that what is in another's mind is of interest, they are developing this capacity.

In the past 20 years there have been many studies of theory of mind in children (e.g., Baron-Cohen et al., 1993). The term has been used by some authors to mean a variety of social knowledge, both verbal and nonverbal, encompassing "general social knowledge." For example, by 10 months of age, children appear to have at least a rudimentary form of theory of mind. In the "Visual Cliff" experimental paradigm (Sorce et al., 1985), a child is placed on a Plexiglas plate that spans two wooden boxes with a space between. The child is placed on one side of the Plexiglas, and his mother is placed on the far side of the second box. When a younger child comes to the "dropoff," he may be fearful and uncertain, but by 10 months of age the child will look to his mother's face. If she displays a fearful or angry face, the child usually will not cross, but when his mother shows a joyful face, he most often will readily cross. Perhaps there was a time millions of years ago when children were temperamentally bolder and were less inhibited in facing cliffs, but if so, the most daring ones fell to the rocks far below, leaving the less daring ones to pass on their "cautious" genes.

Social Knowledge: Folk Psychology and Folk Physics

Understanding that other people have minds that differ from ours is certainly important, but what must we know socially in order to interact with others and socially survive? In its simplest form folk psychology implies the human tendency to view human actions in terms of beliefs, attitudes, and knowledge, whereas objects are viewed in mechanistic and nonmental terms—for example, people have minds and objects do not (e.g., Bennett, 1993; Wellman, 1988). Though folk psychology may sometimes attribute causality to human actions that is simplistic in comparison with psychological concepts, and ignore the complex biopsychosocial underpinnings of why we feel and act as we do, it appears to be a fair description of how we tend to view the world. The question is, how do we come to have these beliefs?

It has been argued, mostly on anecdotal grounds, that even 2-month-old infants appear to respond differently to people than to objects (Brazelton et al., 1974; Trevarthen, 1974). Presented with an object, infants look at it intently, sit up straight, remain relatively still, and alternate between gazing fixedly at the object and glancing away. Presented with people, infants' posture is more relaxed and their movements are smoother. In addition, infants may give a full greeting response to people, but they rarely do so to objects. In the past decade many more studies have established that by 4 years of age, perhaps even by 3 years, children differ in their understanding of people and objects. They talk of "fooling someone," of having dreams, and of "pretending." However, they generally do not attribute motives or theory of mind to objects. These beliefs apparently arise through interactions with people and objects, although adults may also provide cognitive and linguistic knowledge to help them articulate these beliefs. Beyond 3 years of age, children begin to acquire a great wealth of information about other people's motives and how these can be deciphered through the subtle social signals of facial expression, body language, tone of voice, and, of course, what people say, even if this is not always to be trusted. It might be questioned whether there may be a biological propensity to learn this type of information (much of which is nonverbal), similar to our propensity, in childhood, to learn language.

Cognitive knowledge, of the sort represented by the aptitudes and skills measured on standard IQ tests, is equally important. In addition, we need language skills: vocabulary and grammar. "Pragmatic" language skills, representing the "social rules" of language are also important, but they are part of the body of general social knowledge, verbal and nonverbal, discussed earlier.

The body of general social knowledge that we begin to acquire in early childhood, and that we expand greatly in our first 10 years of life, is crucial to our being able to engage in social interactions.

According to Baron-Cohen (1995), to lack this knowledge leads to "mind-blindness." People with mind-blindness cannot predict the behavior of others; worse, they have no implicit nonverbal intuitive sense of what is appropriate in social situations, nor do they have any implicit way of acting to improve their social success. He likens the situation to a game of chess. It is said that chess masters can glance at the pieces on the board and accurately intuit the next best moves. Amateur chess players must try to cognitively work out an approach using a cumbersome and often unsuccessful move-by-move strategy. Humans have the capacity to learn to play social chess with others well beyond an amateur level, even if some do it better than others. What happens if they fail to acquire such a body of social knowledge is discussed in Chapter 8.

Clinical Relevance

Rapid early neurological development is experience-expectant and experience-dependent. Because that experience is interpersonal, the mothering or parenting relationship must be protected, kept as free as possible from stress, bolstered in the event of parental deficiency, and supported so that the parent can provide the milieu in which the infant's brain can develop optimally. The implications for allocations of social resources and for prevention and early intervention are obvious.

Current diagnostic systems describe behaviors and emotional responses that have gone awry. DSM-IV describes it for adults better than for children, and minimally describes the difficulties of very young children and infants. DC 0–3 categorizes disorders of stress modulation, affective regulation, self-regulation, communication, and relationships, but only up to the age of 36 months. What is missing is a diagnostic system that describes what optimal or normal development would look like, describes it from birth to maturity, and, going beyond Axis IV in DSM-IV or Axes II and IV in DC 0–3, describes the fashion in which interpersonal relationships foster mental health or lead to symptomatology.

What early interventions might work? The link between prevention programs, or early stimulation programs, or programs to support parents, and the later well-being of children is tenuous. However, a diagnostic system that is firmly founded in early development, that encompasses the concepts of temperament and social communication, and that characterizes reciprocal behaviors with significant others, appears to be vital to decide if any intervention has been effective in changing the developmental trajectory.

Such a diagnostic system would be consistent with a model of human development that postulates that human infants are endowed with a behavioral capacity to emit social signals involving facial expression and sounds, and that they have a propensity to look to complex social stimuli such as faces, and to monitor sounds within the range of human speech. These propensities, called *affective reciprocity*, are modified through experience to lead to the development of *joint attention*. The subsequent development of a *theory of mind* in the young child may facilitate the development of a body of *social knowledge* that will be necessary for all later human interactions.

REFERENCES

Aitken KKJ & Trevarthen C (1997) Self/other organization in human psychological development. *Dev Psychopathology*, 9(4):653–678.

Allmann JM (1998) *Evolving brains*. New York: Freeman.

Arnstein AFT (1999) Development of the cerebral cortex: XIV. Stress impairs prefrontal cortical function. *J Am Acad Child Adolesc Psychiatry*, 38(2): 220–222.

Baird AA, Gruber SA, Fein DA, Maas LC, Stengard RJ, Renshaw PF, Cohen BM, & Yurgelun-Todd DA (1999) Functional magnetic resonance imaging of facial affect recognition in children and adolescents. *J Am Acad Child Adolesc Psychiatry*, 38(2):195–199.

Baron-Cohen S (1995) *Mindblindness*. Cambridge, MA: MIT Press.

Baron-Cohen S, Tager-Flusberg H, & Cohen D (1993) *Understanding other minds*. New York: Oxford University Press.

Beauchaine T (2001) Vagal tone, development, and Gray's motivational theory: Toward an integrated model of autonomic nervous system functioning in psychopathology. *Dev Psychopathology*, 13(2):183–214.

Beebe B & Lachmann FM (1988) Mother–infant mutual influence and precursors of psychic structure. In A Goldberg (Ed.), *Progress in self psychology* (Vol. 3, p. 325) Hillsdale NJ: Analytic Press.

Bennett SL (Ed.) (1993) *The development of social cognition: The child as psychologist*. New York: Guilford Press.

Berretta S, Robertson HA, & Graybiel AM (1992) Dopamine and glutamate agonists stimulate neuron-specific expression of Fos-like protein in the striatum. *J Neurophysiol*, 68:767–777.

Bertoncini J, Morais J, Bijeljac-Babic R, McAdams S, Peretz I, & Mehler J

(1989) Dichotic perception and laterality in neonates. *Brain Lang*, 37:591–605.

Block J, Block J, & Morrison A (1981) Parental agreement–disagreement on child-rearing orientations and gender-related personality correlates in children. *Child Dev*, 52:965–974.

Brazelton T, Koslowski B, & Main M (1974) The origins of reciprocity: The early mother–infant interaction. In M Lewis & L Rosenblum (Eds.), *The effect of the infant on its caretaker.* New York: Wiley-Interscience.

Brothers L (1989) A biological perspective on empathy. *Am J Psychiatry*, 146:10–19.

Bryan RM Jr. (1990) Cerebral blood flow and energy metabolism during stress. *Am J Physiol*, 259:H269–H280.

Calkins SD, Fox NA, & Marshall TR (1996) Behavioral and physiological antecedents of inhibited and uninhibited behavior. *Child Dev*, 67(2):523–540.

Cherniak C (1995) Neural component placement. *Trends Neurosci*, 18:522–527.

Coplan JD, Andrews MW, Rosenblum LA, Owens MJ, Friedman S, Gorman JM, & Nemeroff CB (1996) Persistent elevations of cerebrospinal fluid concentrations of corticotropin-relasing factor in adult nonhuman primates exposed to early-life stressors: Implications for the pathophysiology of mood and anxiety disorders. *Proc Nat Acad Sci U.S.A.*, 93:1619–1623.

Damasio AR (1994) *Descartes' error: Emotion, reason and the human brain.* New York: Grosset/Putnam.

Davidson RJ & Fox NA (1988) Cerebral asymmetry and emotion: Development and individual differences In DL Molfese & SJ Segalowitz (Eds.), *Brain lateralization in children: Developmental implications* (pp. 191–206). New York: Guilford Press.

Dawson G (1994) Frontal electroencephalographic correlates of individual differences in emotion expression in infants: A brain systems perspective on emotion. In NA Fox (Ed.), The development of emotion regulation: Biological and behavioral considerations. *Monogr So Res Child Dev*, 65(2–3, Serial No, 240):135–151.

Eibl-Eibesfeldt I (1989) *Human ethology.* New York: Aldine de Gruyter.

Emde RN, Polak PR, & Spitz RA (1965) Anaclitic depression in an infant raised in an institution. *J Am Acad Child Adolesc Psychiatry*, 4:545–553.

Field TM, Woodson R, Cohen D, Greenberg R, Garcia R, & Collins K (1983) Discrimination and imitation of facial expressions by term and preterm neonates. *Infant Behav Dev*, 6:485–489.

Fox NA (1991) If it's not left, it's right: Electroencephalogram asymmetry and the development of emotion. *Am Psychol*, 46:843–872.

Fox NA, Calkins SD, & Bell MS (1994) Neural plasticity and development in the first two years of life: Evidence from cognitive and socioemotional domains of research. *Dev Psychopathology*, 6:677–696.

Gage FH, Ray J, & Fisher LJ (1995) Isolation, characterization, and use of stem cells from the CNS. *Annu Rev Neurosci*, 18:159–192.

Goerner S (1995) Chaos, evolution and deep ecology. In R Robertson & A Combs (Eds.), *Chaos theory in psychology and the life sciences* (pp. 17–38). Mahwah, NJ: Erlbaum.

Gorski RA (1999) Development of the cerebral cortex: XV. Sexual differentiation of the central nervous system. *J Am Acad Child Adolesc Psychiatry*, 38(3):344–346.

Greenough WT, Black JE, & Wallace CS (1987) Experience and brain development. *Child Dev*, 58:539–559.

Higley JD, Suomi SJ, & Linnoila M (1991) CSF monoamine metabolite concentrations vary according to age, rearing and sex, and are influenced by the stressor of social separation in rhesus monkeys. *Psychopharamcol*, 103:551–556.

Hubel DH & Wiesel TN (1979) Brain mechanisms of vision. *Sci Am*, 241:150–162.

Hudson JA & Sheffield EG (1998) Déjà vu all over again: Effects of reenactment on toddlers' event memory. *Child Dev*, 69:51–67.

Insel TR & Hulihan TJ (1995) A gender specific mechanism for pair bonding: Oxytocin and partner preference formation in monogamous voles. *Behav Neurosci*, 109(4):782–789.

Insel TR, Preston S, & Winslow JT (1995) Mating in the monogamous male: Behavioral consequences. *Physiol Behav*, 57(4):615–627.

Izard C (1994) Innate and universal facial expressions: Evidence from developmental and cross-cultural research. *Psychol Bull*, 115:288–299.

Jacobsen L & Sapolsky R (1991) The role of the hippocampus in the feedback regulation of the hypothalamic–pituitary–adrenocortical axis. *Endochrinology Rev*, 12:118–134.

Kagan J (2003) Biology, context, and developmental inquiry. *Annu Rev Psychol*, 54:1–23.

Karmiloff-Smith A (1995) Annotation: The extraordinary cognitive journey from fetus through infancy. *J Child Psychol Psychiatry*, 36:1293–1313.

Kaufer D, Friedman A, & Soreq H (1999) The vicious circle of stress and anticholinesterase response. *Neuroscientist*, 5(3):173–183.

Kimberg DV, Loud AV, & Wiener A (1968) Cortisone-induced alterations in mitochondrial function and structure. *J Cell Biol*, 37:63–67.

Kinney HC, Brody BA, Kloman AS, & Gilles FH (1988) Sequence of central nervous system myelination in human infancy: II. Patterns of myelination in autopsied infants. *J Neuropathol Exp Neurol*, 47:217–234.

Kolb B, Forgie M, Gibb R, Gorny G, & Rowntree S (1998) Age, experience, and the changing brain. *Neurosci Biobehav Rev*, 22(2):143–159.

Krubitzer L (1995) The organization of neocortex in mammals: Are species differences really so different? *Trends Neuroscience*, 18:408–417.

Kuhl PK (1991) Perception, cognition, and the ontogenetic and phylogenetic emergence of human speech. In S Brauth, W Hall, & R Dooling (Eds.), *Plasticity of develoment*. Cambridge, MA: MIT Press/Bradford Books.

Kuhl PK, Williams KA, Lacerda F, Stevens KN, & Lindblom B (2000) Linguistic experience alters phonetic perception in infants by six months of age. *Science*, 255:606–608.

LeDoux JE (1992) Emotion and the amygdala. In J. P Aggleton (Ed.), *The amygdala: Neurobiological aspects of emotion, memory and mental dysfunction* (pp. 339–351). New York: Wiley-Liss.

LeDoux JE (1994) Emotion, memory and the brain. *Sci Am*, 270:50–57.

Lieberman AF & Van Horn P (1998) Attachment, trauma and domestic violence. *Child Adolesc Psychiatric Clin North Am*, 7(2):423–443.

Locke JL (1993) *The child's path to spoken language*. Cambridge, MA: Harvard University Press.

Malatesta C & Izard CE (1984). The ontogenesis of human social signals: From biological imperative to symbolic utilization. In N Fox & R Davidson (Eds.), *The psychobiology of affective development* (pp. 161–206). Hillsdale, NJ: Erlbaum.

McHale JP & Rasmussen JL (1998) Coparental and family group-level dynamics during infancy: Early family precursors of child and family functioning during preschool. *Dev Psychopathology*, 10:39–59.

Meltzoff A & Moore M (1977). Imitation of facial and manual gestures by human neonates. *Science*, 198:75–78.

Minuchin P (1985) Families and individual development: Provocations from the field of family therapy. *Child Dev*, 56:289–302.

Mishkin M & Appenzeller T (1987) The anatomy of memory. *Sci Am*, 256:80–89.

Morell V (1999) Ecology returns to speciation studies. *Science*, 284:2106–2108.

Newcomer JW, Selke GS, Melson AK, Hershey T, Craft S, Richards K, & Alderson AL (1999) Decreased memory performance in healthy humans induced by stress-level cortisol treatment. *Arch Gen Psychiatry*, 56:527–553.

Novelli A, Reilly JA, Lysko PG, & Henneberry RC (1988) Glutamate becomes neurotoxic via the N-methyl-D-aspartate receptor when intracellular energy levels are reduced. *Brain Res*, 451:205–212.

Ockleford EM, Vince MA, Layton C, Reader MR (1988) Responses of neonates to parents' and others' voices. *Early Hum Dev*, 18(1):27–36.

Perry DB, Pollard RA, Blakley TL, Maker WL, & Vigilante D (1995) Childhood trauma: The neurobiology of adaptation and "use-dependent" development of the brain: How states become traits. *Infant Ment Health J*, 16:271–291.

Plutchik R (1980). *Emotion—A psychoevolutionary synthesis*. New York: Harper & Row.

Porges SW (1995) Orienting in a defensive world: Mammalian modifications of our evolutionary heritage: A polyvagal theory. *Psychophysiology*, 32:301–318.

Porges SW, Doussard-Roosevelt JA, & Maiti AK (1994) Vagal tone and the physiological regulation of emotion. *Monog Soc Res Child Dev*, 59:167–186.

Purves D & LaMantia AS (1990) Construction of modular circuits in the mammalian brain. *Cold Spring Harbor Symp Quant Biol*, LV:445–452.

Rodrigues SM, Schafe GE, & LeDoux JE (2004) Molecular mechanisms underlying emotional learning and memory in the lateral amygdala. *Neuron*, 44:75–91.

Rogan MT & LeDoux JE (1996) Emotion: Systems, cells, synaptic plasticity. *Cell*, 85:469–475.

Sackett G (1966) Monkeys reared in isolation with pictures as visual input: Evidence for an innate releasing mechanism. *Science*, 154:1468–1473.

Sapolsky R (1992) *Stress, the aging brain and the mechanisms of neuron death*. Cambridge, MA: MIT Press.

Sapolsky R (2000) Glucocorticoids and hippocampal atrophy in neuropsychiatric disorders. *Arch Gen Psychiatry*, 57:925–934.

Sapolsky RM (2004) Is impaired neurogenesis relevant to the affective symptoms of depression? *Biol Psychiatry*, 56:137–139.

Sapolsky RM, Krey LC, & McEwen BS (1986) The neuroendochrinology of stress and aging: The glucocorticoid cascade hypothesis. *Endocrinology Rev*, 7:284-310.

Scaife M & Bruner J (1975) The capacity for joint visual attention in the infant. *Nature*, 253:265–266.

Schneider ML, Roughton RC, Koehler AJ, & Lubach GR (1999) Growth and development following prenatal stress exposure in primates: An examination of ontogenetic vulnerability. *Child Dev*, 70(2):263–536.

Schore AN (1997) Early organization of the nonlinear right brain and development of a predisposition to psychiatric disorders. *Dev Psychopathology*, 9(4):595–632.

Snyder EY (1998) Neural stem-like cells: Developmental lessons with therapeutic potential. *Neuroscientist*, 4(6):408–425.

Sorce J, Emde R, Campos J, & Klinnert M (1985) Maternal emotional signaling: Its effect on the visual cliff behavior of 1-year olds. *Dev Psychol*, 21:195–200.

Spinelli DN (1987) Plasticity triggering experiences, nature, and the dual genesis of brain structure and function. In N Guzenhauser (Ed.), *Infant stimulation: For whom, what kind, when, and how much?* Skillman, NJ: Johnson & Johnson.

Spitz R (1945) Hospitalism: An inquiry into the genesis of psychiatric conditions in early childhood. *Psychoanal Study Child*, 1:53.

Stern D (1977) *The first relationship*. Cambridge, MA: Harvard University Press.

Trevarthen C (1974) Conversation with a two-month old. *New Scientist*, 896:230–235.

Tronick EZ (1989) Emotions and emotional communications in infants. *Am Psychol*, 44:112–119.

Tuszynski MH (1998) Gene therapy: Applications to the neurosciences and to neurological disease. *Neuroscientist*, 4(6):398–407.

Vecera S & Johnson M (1995) Eye gaze detection and the cortical processing of faces: Evidence from infants and adults. *Vis Cogn*, 2:101–129.

Waddington VCH (1966). *Principles of development and differentiation*. New York: Macmillan.

Wang L & Pitts DK (1994) Postnatal development of mesoaccumbens dopamine neurons in the rat: Electrophysiological studies. *Dev Brain Res*, 79:19–28.

Weinstock M (1996) Does prenatal stress impair coping and regulation of hypothalamic–pituitary–adrenal axis? *Neurosci Biobehav Rev*, 21(1):1–10.

Wellman HW (1988) *The child's theory of mind*. Cambridge, MA: MIT Press.

Werner E (1995) Resilience in development *Curr Dir Psychol Sci*, 4:81–84.

Winnicott DW (1990) *The maturational process and the facilitating environment*. London: Karnac Books and the Institute of Psychoanalysis.

Woodward SA, McManis MH, Kagan J, Deldin P, Snidman N, Lewis M, & Kahn V (2001, July) Infant temperament and the brainstem auditory evoked response in later childhood. *Dev Psychol*, 37(4):533–538.

Zahn-Waxler C, Radke-Yarrow M, Wagner E, & Chapman M (1992) Development of concern for others. *Dev Psychol*, 126–136.

CHAPTER 4

A Developmental Evolutionary Perspective on Two Anxiety Disorders

DANIEL S. PINE *and* THEODORE SHAPIRO

Clinical advances in psychiatry have lagged in the face of basic science advances, owing to difficulties in working with descriptive categories uncertainly linked to biological underpinnings. Nowhere is the need for a melding of basic and clinical science more salient than in the study of anxiety. Conceptualizations of anxiety have taxed psychiatric wisdom because of difficulties in clearly distinguishing normal from pathological anxiety and in understanding interactions between psychosocial and biological factors. Evolutionary psychobiology holds the hope of smoothing the integration of basic and clinical science (McGuire & Troisi, 1998, Neese & Williams, 1994). Historically, thinkers from Freud on have taken an evolutionary view of anxiety as an emergency emotion that aids adaptation.

Freud's earliest view of anxiety was colored by his belief that drives were inhibited by social constraints, preventing discharge (Freud, 1962). The energy was transformed into "actual" anxiety, conceptualized as a biological threshold phenomenon onto which psychoneuroses were grafted and then psychologically analyzed. This theory brought Freud to a radical evolutionary construct first voiced by Darwin (1998). Anxiety neuroses were themselves viewed as the evolutionary remnants of prehistoric human experiences. The phenomenological properties of an anxiety attack were thought to represent replays of a prior conflicted reminiscence.

Central themes in current research resemble those put forth by Freud in 1926, stimulating Bowlby's wide-ranging modifications of Freudian theory (Bowlby, 1969). This theory emphasized the dual nature of human anxiety, noting a physiological, possibly subcortical component, intrinsic to the organism, and a psychological component, arising during development with cortical maturation. Although some current theoreticians emphasize subcortical contributions to anxiety (Graeff, 1997; Graeff et al., 1997; Gray & McNaughton, 1996; LeDoux, 1996; Panksepp, 1998), others place equally strong emphasis on cortically based cognitive mediation of subcortical anxiety-related processes (Barlow, 1988). As a corollary to emphasizing dual roles for higher and more primitive brain regions, Freud stressed the developmental aspects of anxiety, refusing to equate the early physiologic anlage of anxiety with mature anxiety (Freud, 1959). Instead, he suggested that although anxiety can always be seen as a response to perceived danger, the response is elicited by threats of different salience at each developmental stage. This ontogenetic array of perceived threats was summarized in the epigraph that early fear of the threat of the loss of the mother, as necessary caretaker, is in maturity represented as the threat of the psychological loss of the love of the mother. These views presaged modern theoreticians' emphasis on the importance of developmental processes in the genesis of clinical anxiety disorders (Barlow, 1988; Klein, 1993).

Whereas many modern theories of anxiety involve components of evolutionary theory (Bowlby, 1969; Freud, 1959; Gilbert, 2001; Gray & McNaughton, 1996; Klein, 1993, 1995; Marks, 1987; Nesse, 1999), few theories attempt to explain why humans are susceptible to specific illnesses through explicit reliance on the principles of evolution. Such genuinely evolutionary theories attempt to integrate basic and clinical research by generating testable hypotheses about pathophysiology for specific illnesses (McGuire & Troisi, 1998; Neese & Williams, 1994). For example, Sapolsky (1992, 2000) suggests that although our body's stress response system facilitated survival for our ancestors, it left our hippocampus vulnerable to insults that may predispose our species to major depression and

Alzheimer's disease. This theory produced advances in the understanding of stress physiology and generated hypotheses about pre vention of depression (Sapolsky, 2004). We propose a similar evolutionary theory for anxiety disorders. We first review general principles that inform the current evolutionary theory in light of recent research on the biology and developmental plasticity of fear responses. We then apply evolutionary theory to two conditions, social phobia and panic disorder, for which there is a wealth of relevant research.

GENERAL PRINCIPLES

Neural Circuits Involved in Anxiety

The most current neuroscientific research suggests that separate but interrelated brain circuits play distinct roles in mediating an organism's response to various forms of danger (Graeff, 1997; Graeff et al., 1997; Gray & McNaughton, 1996; LeDoux, 1996; Panksepp, 1998). Considerable work in this area focuses on circuits mediating organisms' response to discrete conditioned fear stimuli. In fear conditioning experiments, an explicit neutral cue stimulus, such as a tone or a light, is paired with an aversive unconditioned stimulus, such as a shock (LeDoux, 1996). Physiological responses to formerly neutral stimuli change after conditioning, producing a brain state labeled "conditioned fear," which results from neural modifications in an amygdala-based circuit. Circuits based in the cortex, hippocampus, or other limbic structures are also activated by visualization of the context, allowing higher-order processes to impact on amygdala-based processes (LeDoux, 1996; McNish et al., 1997). Hence, a subcortical substrate facilitates arousal in the face of potential adversity. With maturation of relevant brain regions, psychological components of anticipation and dread are expected to play increasingly prominent roles in mediating organisms' response to danger cues.

The conditioned fear response to an explicit cue can be contrasted with the reaction to other danger-related stimuli, such as dangerous contexts or overtly threatening scenarios. Unconditioned, contextually conditioned, and cue-specific conditioned fear responses can each be differentiated on neuroanatomical and pharmacological grounds (Davis 1997; Graeff, 1997; Graeff et al., 1997; Gray & McNaughton, 1996; LeDoux, 1996; McNish et al., 1997; Panksepp, 1998; Walker & Davis, 1997). As such, each response may potentially model unique aspects of human anxiety. For example, as outlined in the following paragraph, systems related to cue-specific conditioned fear may play a role in phobias, and systems related to unconditioned fear may play a role in disorders related to spontaneous panic attacks.

Clinical studies also implicate a network of distinct fear-relevant circuits in various forms of anxiety. Although neuroimaging and lesion studies suggest involvement of the human amygdala in cue-specific fear conditioning (Bechara et al., 1995; Furmark et al., 1997; LaBar et al., 1998), imaging studies emphasize the role of extra-amygdala structures in other forms of anxiety (Peterson & Klein, 1997; Rauch et al., 1997). Pharmacological studies also emphasize a role for different circuits in various aspects of anxiety. Hence, medications that treat panic disorder are seen as acting via brain systems intimately tied to innate or immediately present danger, whereas medications that treat generalized anxiety disorder may act via other brain systems that show stronger associations with less direct or immediate danger (Bowlby, 1969; Graeff, 1997; Graeff et al., 1997). Finally, ethology also implicates multiple fear circuits in anxiety. Mammals never in contact with natural predators respond with fear when they are presented, and humans show fear of snakes and heights, never having been conditioned (Marks, 1987; Neese & Williams, 1994).

Human alarm systems are thought to develop from the systems of lower mammals. The basic operations of these systems are evolutionarily conserved, in that the systems involve primitive portions of the brain, produce similar effects on peripheral physiology across species, and are similarly moderated by chemical perturbations (Graeff, 1997; Graeff et al., 1997; Gray & McNaughton, 1996; LeDoux, 1996; Panksepp, 1998). The systems possess obvious survival value, in that organisms without such systems would face risk from separation and predators.

Given that distinct brain circuits are implicated in distinct aspects of anxiety, different evolutionary pressures are thought to have shaped a distinct set of circuits, possibly producing variability in the regulation of each circuit. There is relatively little genetic variability in traits carrying a strong selective advantage, for if a trait is highly adaptive, the forces of natural selection create population homogeneity. Because genes from individuals with frank defects in alarm systems are unlikely to propagate, individual differences in anxiety are more likely to result from relatively subtle perturbations of alarm circuits. For example, such perturbations could involve abnormalities in input systems to circuits underlying conditioned, contextual, or unconditioned fears; hypersensitivity in limbic structures essential to the process of conditioned fear; or abnormalities in higher brain centers that modulate subcortical fear circuits. These perturbations may relate to plasticity in anxiety-related circuitry, as conceptualized from developmental, neural, and psychological perspectives.

Plasticity: Behavioral and Brain Systems

Current theories of chronic psychiatric disorders emphasize developmental psychopathological perspectives. Evolutionary theories of anxiety benefit from such perspectives, if one accepts the developmental principle that there is a changing ontogenetic field in which the context of the signal function of anxiety changes over the lifespan. Evidence from developmental research on behavioral, psychological, and neural systems supports this view.

Behavioral Plasticity: Pathology as Failure of Adaptive Processes

From the behavioral perspective, plasticity can be viewed as the ability to adjust behavior to changing life circumstances. As such changes are a vital part of childhood, many forms of childhood psychopathology can be viewed as failures of behavioral plasticity or as distortions of the adaptive developmental process. For example, separation anxiety is normal in young children as it facilitates attachment; it is considered a sign of pathology only when it persists into latency or disrupts social adaptation (Shapiro & Jegede, 1973). Thus, separation anxiety disorder represents an anachronistic developmental failure in adaptation where new demands are met with the apprehension appropriate to situations in which a caretaker is needed for survival.

Although this developmental perspective is most clearly illustrated for separation anxiety disorder, it can be similarly applied to other anxiety disorders. The earliest epidemiological investigations note anxiety and fear to be a normal part of childhood (Lapouse & Monk, 1958). Subsequent studies have been plagued by the difficulty in distinguishing common, developmentally appropriate forms of anxiety from pathological anxiety (Costello & Angold, 1995; Pine 1997). Although impairment ratings aid in distinguishing "caseness" from normal variation, there is tremendous variation in impairment thresholds across studies, leading to a fivefold variation in prevalence estimates for childhood anxiety disorders in the most current studies (Costello & Angold, 1995; Pine, 1997; Verhulst et al., 1997). If relatively liberal impairment thresholds are used, the majority of adult anxiety, as well as affective disorders, are presaged by childhood anxiety, though most childhood anxiety disorders studied prospectively prove to be transient (Pine et al., 1998a). These findings lead to a view of anxiety disorders as pathologies in developmental processes. There are relatively high rates of anxiety and fear during childhood which typically recede with age. Anxiety disorders may result from failures in development, producing maladaptive regulation of fear responses.

Short- and Long-Term Plasticity in Fear-Relevant Circuitry

Given the view of anxiety disorders as failures in adaptive processes, variations in anxiety, both between individuals and in the same individual over time, may be attributed to developmental variation. Such developmental differences, in turn, may arise from plastic changes in neural systems that facilitate an organism's response to danger.

Systems mediating fear conditioning to explicit cues exhibit both short- and long-term plasticity. Fear conditioning results from short-term changes in amygdala neurons, mediated by glutamate (Davis, 1997; LeDoux, 1996; McNish et al., 1997; Panksepp, 1998; Walker & Davis, 1997). Long-term plasticity in the amygdala can be facilitated by neurons relying on corticotropin-releasing factor (CRF) as a neurotransmitter. Severe adversity associated with CRF stimulation of the amygdala may prime the fear-conditioning circuit during development, facilitating glutamate-based plasticity possibly by altering underlying genetic processes (Rosen & Schulkin, 1998).

Similarly, neural circuits mediating anxiety associated with attachment and separation behaviors exhibit both short- and long-term plasticity. Ultrasonic distress vocalization and related protest behaviors in mammals serve to maintain the attachment of mother–infant pair-bonds, which, in turn, form the basis for later separation, independent adult action, and procreative aims of a species (Panksepp, 1998). The survival value of attachment-oriented behaviors are complemented by the distress signal and associated anxiety that mark attempts to recapture the bond between mother and infant. Insel's (1977) work with prairie voles demonstrates the key role of the nonapeptides, oxytocin and vasopressin, in the short-term plasticity of attachment behaviors. These compounds control acute changes in adult pair-bonding, monogamy, and paternal behavior. Close cousins, the montane voles, differing in only one amino acid in their nonapeptides, show none of the affiliative, monogamous, or caretaking roles of the prairie cousins. Parallel work examines long-term plasticity in circuits effected by attachment behaviors. Variations in maternal behavior produce hippocampally mediated changes in the stress response of rodent pups that persist throughout the life of an organism (Francis et al., 1996; Liu et al., 1997; Meany et al., 1993).

Although studies in lower mammals emphasize the role of hippocampal or amygdala-based plasticity, a more prominent role for cortical plasticity may be expected in fear among primates. Bowlby (1969) argued that protest signals become increasingly important for the maintenance of mother–brood mutuality as phylogenetic complexity increases. Darwin (1998) similarly noted that small primate broods necessitate longer periods of caretaking. Although the neurochemical regulation of separation anxiety appears similar in primates and rodents (Kalin, 1993; Panksepp, 1998; Panksepp et al., 1992), longer caretaking coupled with increasing cortical complexity allows for psychological components to play increasingly prominent roles in primate attachment.

Schneirla (Schneirla & Rosenblatt, 1961) first drew the distinction between biosocial and psychosocial organization, demonstrating that early experience supersedes biosocial cues once infancy attachment is completed. These internalized patterns shape later social behavior, facilitating survival. Thus, among primates, cortical perception of dangerous social situations may play a unique role in mediating emotional states associated with subcortically based change. Such a unique role might be expected in light of the species-typical complex web of social relationships that encourages the manipulation of mental scenarios to anticipate the reactions of conspecifics. Among primates, the tie to the mother is dependent on an array of "component instincts" released by early experience (Bowlby, 1969; Harlow et al., 1973). Manipulations of the rearing environment may alter inborn response systems, which in turn may disrupt plasticity in cortical circuits essential for social adjustment and the control of fear-relevant behaviors. Poorly mothered primates show both abnormalities in fear-relevant behaviors as well as an inability to assume the necessary social behaviors for coitus and species survival (Coplan et al., 1995). Similarly, among humans, a child's response to separation in the classic "strange situation" paradigm (Ainsworth et al., 1978) predicts anxiety symptoms in adolescence, despite imprecision in attachment classification (Warren et al., 1997). Contrariwise, the meaning of the infant to the mother prior to birth alter attachment measured at 14–20 months (Fonagy & Steele, 1991).

In summary, anxiety disorders can be seen as failures in adaptive processes. Such adaptive processes are thought to involve changes in cortical and subcortical systems. Studies with lower mammals show that life experiences impinge on evolutionarily adaptive subcortical systems to create differences in the predilection to experience fear and anxiety. Studies with primates suggest that life experiences might also change adaptive cortical systems, further contributing to differences in later anxiety-related behavior. As a result, the current theories emphasize the role of developmental plasticity in evolutionarily adaptive biological systems.

EVOLUTIONARY PERSPECTIVES
ON TWO ANXIETY DISORDERS

Anxiety disorders are thought to arise from vulnerabilities in specific fear-relevant systems. These vulnerabilities are a by-product of selective forces' effects on particular behavioral, psychological, and biological systems characteristic of each specific anxiety disorder. Although each anxiety disorder is presumably the by-product of vulnerabilities in some core alarm system, there is relatively firm evidence to support the view of anxiety disorders as a family of distinct conditions. These data include the unique phenomenology, family history, treatment, course, and biology of each disorder. For example, obsessive–compulsive disorder shows a unique association with basal ganglia pathology (Peterson & Klein, 1997). Panic disorder shows a unique association with respiratory dysfunction (Klein, 1993; Papp et al., 1997). With social phobia, there is evidence of a unique developmental course, treatment response pattern, family profile, and biological correlates (Pine et al., 1998b, 1998c). We discuss evolutionary theories for two anxiety disorders, social phobia and separation anxiety disorder, for which there is a wealth of relevant developmental, neuroscientific research.

As demonstrated by Sapolsky (1992), useful evolutionary theories must go beyond post hoc rationalizations and generate hypotheses that change the conceptualization of a syndrome. Accordingly, we offer evolutionary theories for social phobia and panic disorder that generate explicit testable hypotheses. Given the view of these anxiety disorders as developmental conditions, hypotheses involve predictions concerning the relationship between child and adult disorders. Each disorder is first discussed within the context of existing developmental, clinical psychobiological data and within the context of evolutionary theory. Developmental hypotheses are then put forth, with respect to behavioral and biological aspects of each condition.

Social Phobia

Social phobia is thought to involve the circuitry of fear conditioning. An amygdala-based circuit may be oversensitive to signals that arise in social interchanges, such as facial expressions (LeDoux, 1996). Given primates' increased dependency on social relationships for survival, circuitry that sensitizes individuals to potentially dangerous social scenarios would carry evolutionary advantages. Recent functional imaging data confirm the involvement of the fear-conditioning circuit in social perception: the amygdala responds selectively to fearful faces, even when presented below the level of conscious perception (Breiter et al., 1996; Whalen et al., 1998). Moreover, preliminary evidence suggests that adults with social phobia show enhanced sensitivity in their amygdala for facial displays of emotion (Birbaumer et al., 1998).

Social phobia also is unique from the developmental perspective. Many adults report preteen onset of social phobia, whereas panic and generalized anxiety disorders typically arise after puberty (Pine, 1997; Schneier et al., 1992). Prospective studies confirm these findings in all three anxiety disorders, while also revealing marked specificity in the course of social phobia as distinct from the other anxiety disorders (Pine et al., 1998a). Kagan and colleagues (1988) note a biological predisposition for shyness as a temperamental trait in a sizable minority of preschool children. Such children exhibit signs of behavioral inhibition, the tendency to withdraw from novelty, particularly social novelty. Like social phobia, this behavioral pattern is thought to result from activity in the amygdala-based fear circuit. Although the precise relationship between behavioral inhibition and individual childhood anxiety disorders remains a matter of dispute, there is evidence of a specific tie with social phobia (Kagan, 1997).

Neuroscientific and developmental data suggest that social phobia may result from a perturbation in the sensitivity of the fear circuit, as it responds to cues of potentially hostile social scenarios (Birbaumer et al., 1998; Breiter et al., 1996; Kagan, 1997; Kagan et al., 1988; Schneier et al., 1992; Whalen et al., 1998). Based on developmental data, such hypersensitivity is expected to arise early in life, preceding overt manifestation of the disorder (Kagan, 1997; Kagan et al., 1988). From the evolutionary standpoint, the propensity for our species to develop social phobia may derive from the selective advantage conveyed to ancestors who were particularly sensitive to cues of social hostility (Ohman, 1986). Although currently observable remnants of this selective advantage may not be obvious, they may be observable where predators abound. Even now, humans develop amid the dangers of war zones and ghettos. Recently emerging literature on conduct disorder reveals the potential survival value of an amygdala-based brain circuit responsive to social displeasure in some contexts.

The pattern of repeated aggressive and rule-violating behavior of conduct disorder is particularly common among children living under social duress. Conduct disorder often persists and sometimes develops into antisocial personality disorder (Moffitt, 1993). Anxiety and conduct disorders frequently co-occur (Bird et al., 1993), but there is controversy about whether comorbid anxiety disorders signal a more benign or malignant form of conduct disorder (Brennan & Raine, 1997; Graham & Rutter, 1973; Ialongo et al., 1996; Kerr et al., 1997; Mitchell & Rosa, 1981; Raine, 1993; Raine et al., 1998). If social phobia results from specific enhanced sensitivity for social cues in an evolutionary adaptive, developmentally preserved circuit, such enhanced sensitivity might alert children with conduct disorder to social pressures, which effectively moderates behavior. Therefore, one might predict that childhood social phobia, but not other forms of anxiety, would signal a more benign course away from conduct disorder.

There is evidence to support this view. Kerr and colleagues (1997) found that symptoms of behavioral inhibition predict a relatively transient course for aggressive symptoms in children. Raine (Raine, 1993; Raine et al., 1998) also showed that enhanced sensitivity for fear conditioning predicted transient symptoms of aggression. Recent data extend these findings to symptom ratings of both social phobia and conduct disorder (Pine et al., 2000). Specifically, symptoms of social phobia, but not other anxiety disorders, were shown to predict a more transient course of conduct disorder symptoms. Bowlby and others' earliest studies showed that the most characteristic malignant outcome of nonattached preschoolers was affectionless criminality without overt anxiety (Bowlby, 1969).

This evolutionary view of social phobia also generates more specific predictions in terms of neural physiology. For example, one might predict that increased sensitivity of the amygdala-based fear circuit to social cues, as assessed using functional magnetic resonance imaging (fMRI), also predicts a more benign course for conduct disorder. Similarly, increased sensitivity to social cues in young inhibited or even asymptomatic children might predict the onset of social phobia. In summary, evolutionary theory provides a hypothesis that social phobia might result from adaptive advantages conferred by the fear circuit's activation when there are cues from hostile social surrounds. Such a theory might suggest survival of this characteristic in the population through its ability to adaptively influence behavior in some situations, as hypothesized for conduct disorder. Finally, such a theory generates a set of specific, testable hypotheses that may change conceptualizations of social phobia and enhance understandings of pathophysiology.

Panic Disorder

As the link between panic disorder and respiration stands as one of the best-replicated findings in the psychiatric literature, virtually all pathophysiological theories recognize the salience of respiratory factors (Barlow, 1988; Goddard & Charney, 1997; Graeff, 1997; Graeff et al., 1997; Gray & McNaughton, 1996; Klein, 1993; LeDoux, 1996; Panksepp, 1998). Situations, such as respiratory illness or near drowning, that produce smothering are specifically associated with the development of panic but not other anxiety disorders (Bouwer & Stein, 1997). Conversely, panic disorder in healthy untraumatized individuals is associated with "CO_2 hypersensitivity," observable as enhanced anxiety, dyspnea, and respiratory rate responses to CO_2 or other respiratory challenges (Klein, 1995; Papp et al., 1997; Pine et al., 1998c).

The cause of this association remains an area of intense debate. Klein (1993) provides an essentially evolutionary perspective, viewing the panic attack as an alarm reaction that developed to alert organisms to cues of impending suffocation. Other biological theories view respiratory manifestations as a downstream reflection of prefrontal or limbic structure's effects on lower respiratory centers (Davis, 1997; Goddard & Charney, 1997; LeDoux, 1996). Cognitive theories emphasize the role of mental distortions related to hypersensitivity to somatic respiratory cues, social stress, or loss of control (Barlow, 1988; Marks, 1987). Psychodynamic views also focus on the misapprehension of body sensations and add the idea of fear of loss of protection shown by the expression of aggression and potential protest toward the perceived caretaker. Despite debate on specifics, there is clear consensus across the various theories on two key points that inform the current theory. Namely, the spontaneous panic attack involves a prominent respiratory component and represents an adult phenomenon with childhood antecedents. The current theory places these points within the context of evolutionary psychobiology.

Spontaneous panic attacks exhibit very low rates before puberty, with an initiation, steady rise, and eventual peak from puberty through early adulthood (Pine, 1997; Pine et al., 1998a). Few adolescents who suffer spontaneous panic attacks develop full-blown panic disorder, which has a median age of onset in the 20s (Pine et al., 1998c). Nevertheless, most adults with panic disorder had suffered from a childhood anxiety disorder or an adolescent panic attack (Klein, 1995; Pine et al., 1998a). Hence, panic disorder, like social phobia, might result from failure in adaptive processes, as signaled by various forms of anxiety during childhood.

The association between separation anxiety and panic disorders has sparked particular interest. Despite some controversy, the weight of the evidence supports an association between the two conditions. From the neurobiological perspective, the pharmacology and neuroanatomy of separation reactions in animals bears similarity to the pharmacology of human spontaneous panic (Panksepp, 1998; Panksepp et al., 1992). Both conditions can be differentiated on pharmacological and anatomical grounds from other forms of fear. From the clinical perspective, separation anxiety disorder identifies a particularly familial form of panic disorder, with an early age of onset (Battaglia et al., 1995). Such early-onset panic disorder is more familial and more closely tied to the spontaneous panic attack, which, in turn, is most closely tied to respiratory factors (Briggs et al., 1993; Goldstein et al., 1994). Children of parents with panic disorder exhibit high rates of separation anxiety, also suggesting a familial and possibly genetic association (Capps et al., 1996; Klein, 1995). Adults with panic disorder retrospectively report high rates of separation anxiety disorder, and prospectively followed children with separation anxiety disorder exhibit high rates of panic as adults (Klein, 1995; Pine et al., 1998a). Difficulty with separation experiences among adults can presage the development of panic attacks, occurring either naturally (Brown et al., 1996) or in the laboratory (Carter et al., 1995). Finally, children with separation anxiety disorder exhibit many of the classic respiratory manifestations seen in adults with panic disorder (Pine et al., 1997, 1998b).

The data on the developmental course of spontaneous panic attacks and on the relationships between panic attacks, respiration, and separation anxiety form the basis for the current evolutionary theory. This theory suggests that both the spontaneous panic attack and separation anxiety disorder involve perturbations in brain circuits centrally involved in respiratory control. This may account for the prominent role of vocalization in separation anxiety among both animals and humans. From a developmental, evolutionary standpoint, the current theory posits a pubertal change in the common circuitry that mediates separation anxiety before puberty and panic reactions after puberty. Evolutionarily, a change in this circuit was ontogenetically adaptive for our ancestors in the face of changing environmental demands at puberty. These demands required different forms of respiratory control as the need for vocalizations to maintain physical attachment diminished. Conversely, as humans spent decreasing amounts of time in proximity to caretakers, the respiratory system was refined to facilitate rapid physical exertion upon exposure to unexpectedly dangerous situations, including suffocation. Hence, changes in the regulation of separation, respiration, and underlying panic circuitry facilitate successful navigation of individuation, self-care, and changing socioenvironmental pressures around puberty. The adaptive plasticity in this circuit, however, is hypothesized to leave our species vulnerable for separation anxiety disorder before puberty and spontaneous panic attacks after puberty.

This theory generates a number of testable hypotheses, some of which have already received preliminary support. First, children with separation anxiety disorder, like adults with panic disorder, are expected to exhibit enhanced sensitivity to respiratory stimulants, manifested both in terms of dyspnea complaints and physiology. Such enhanced sensitivity is a by-product of plasticity in systems mediating both separation anxiety and panic. Preliminary data from our group are consistent with this hypothesis (Pine et al., 1997, 1998c). Second, respiratory sensitivity to cues of suffocation should become increasingly prominent as children with separation anxiety disorder approach puberty, reflecting the evolutionary advantage of adapting the respiratory system for prompt mobilization. Such alterations in puberty facilitate biological responses to circumstances that require sudden mobilization of the respiratory system designed to escape predators, engage in combat for sexual primacy, or elude suffocating circumstances. However, overpriming may result in a propensity for panic attacks in our species. Third, such changes in respiration will be paralleled by changes in other biological systems related to a diminution in separation anxiety. For example, one might expect changes in the coupling between the hypothalamic–pituitary–adrenal (HPA) axis and the respiratory system, as the HPA axis and the respiratory system are coactivated during separation (Panksepp et al., 1992), whereas panic is associated with isolated respiratory activation (Klein, 1993). Although respiratory mobilization is part of both separation anxiety and panic, HPA activation is adaptive for separation anxiety but maladaptive in suffocation (Klein, 1993).

Finally, respiratory and HPA axis change will be tied to social changes at puberty, given that the relevant circuitry is thought to facilitate adaptation to socioenvironmental challenges at puberty. Viewed from a psychological perspective, the acute body consciousness of pubertal adolescents possessing an underlying subcortical vulnerability may promote maladaptive overinterpretation of bodily sensations. This, in turn, may be coupled with the generation of anxiety from psychological conflicts, as judged by a relatively socially immature organism. The introduction of adolescence as a psychosocial phase in development places the procreatively competent postpubertal human in a position where she is capable of reproduction but societally inhibited, leading to anxiety about misconstruals of social signals and intrapsychic desires.

In summary, there are intimate connections between respiration, spontaneous panic, and separation anxiety. From a developmental, neuroscientific, and family-genetic perspective, separation anxiety disorder presages an increased risk for spontaneous panic arising during puberty. From an evolutionary perspective, a common biological system is involved in the regulation of separation reactions, respiration, and panic. Developmental changes in this system facilitate the navigation of puberty but also expose our species to the risk for spontaneous panic.

CONCLUSIONS

This chapter illustrates the utility of evolutionary theory in synthesizing the rapidly accumulating body of knowledge in neuroscience and clinical psychiatry. An evolutionary view of anxiety is by no means new, as debate on the primary role of physiological versus psychological factors has characterized evolutionarily based theories arising throughout the century. The current essay adds developmental and neuroscientific perspectives to this debate. Earlier principles are placed within a developmental context, calling attention to the well-documented plasticity in fear-related behaviors and associated neural circuits. Moreover, such developmental views are integrated with current knowledge on the distinctions among fear-relevant circuits that mediate responses to various forms of danger. Most significant, this chapter applies evolutionary theory to two anxiety disorders, social phobia and panic disorder, demonstrating that such a view generates a new set of testable hypotheses that may advance our understanding of pathophysiology. As noted by Neese and Williams (1994), the true value of an evolutionary theory lies not in proof of its veracity, as such proof is not possible, but in the theory's ability to synthesize data in a manner that generates testable hypotheses concerning pathophysiology. In short, the evolutionary view provides a rational explanation of the segregation of two anxiety syndromes, linking the phenomenology to specific physiological evolutionarily determined precursors.

REFERENCES

Ainsworth M, Blehar MC, Waters E, & Wall S (1978) *Patterns of attachment: A psychological study of the strange situation.* Hillsdale, NJ: Erlbaum.
Barlow DH (1988) *Anxiety and its disorders: The nature and treatment of anxiety and panic.* New York: Guilford Press.
Battaglia M, Bertella S, Politi E, Bernardeschi L, Perna G, Gabriele A, &

Bellodi L (1995) Age at onset of panic disorder: Influence of familial liability to the disease and of childhood separation anxiety disorder. Am J Psychiatry, 152:1362–1364.

Bechara A, Tranel D, Damasio H, Adolphs R, Rockland C, & Damasio AR (1995) Double dissociation of conditioning and declarative knowledge relative to the amygdala and hippocampus in humans. Science, 269:1115–1118.

Birbaumer N, Grodd W, Diedrich O, Klose U, Erb M, Lotze M, Schneider F, Weiss U, & Flor H (1998) fMRI reveals amygdala activation to human faces in social phobics. NeuroReport, 9:1223–1226.

Bird HR, Gould MS, & Staghezza BM (1993) Patterns of diagnostic comorbidity in a community sample of children aged 9 through 16 years. J Am Acad Child Adolesc Psychiatry, 32:361–368.

Bouwer C & Stein DJ (1997) Association of panic disorder with a history of traumatic suffocation. Am J Psychiatry, 154:1566–1567.

Bowlby J (1969) Attachment and loss (Vol. 1). New York: Basic Books.

Breiter HC, Etcoff JL, Whalen PJ, Kennedy WA, Rauch SL, Buckner RL, Strauss MM, Hyman SE, & Rosen BR (1996) Response and habituation of the human amygdala during visual processing of facial expression. Neuron, 17:875–887.

Brennan PA & Raine A (1997) Biosocial bases of antisocial behavior: Psychophysiological, neurological, and cognitive factors. Clin Psychol Rev, 17:589–604.

Briggs AC, Stretch DD, & Brandon S (1993) Subtyping of panic disorder by symptom profile. Br J Psychiatry, 163:201–209.

Brown GW, Harris TO, & Eales MJ (1996) Social factors and comorbidity of depressive and anxiety disorders. Br J Psychiatry Suppl, 30:50–57.

Capps L, Sigman M, Sena R, Henker B, & Whalen C (1996) Fear, anxiety and perceived control in children of agoraphobic parents. J Child Psychol Psychiatry, 37:445–452.

Carter MM, Hollan SD, Carson R, & Shelton RC (1995) Effects of a safe person on induced distress following a biological challenge in panic disorder with agorophobia. J Abnorm Psychol, 104:156–161.

Coplan JD, Rosenblum LA, & Gorman JM (1995) Primate models of anxiety. Longitudinal perspectives. Psychiatr Clin North Am, 18:727–743.

Costello EJ & Angold A (1995) Epidemiology. In JS March (Ed.), Anxiety disorders in children and adolescents (pp. 109–124). New York, Guilford Press.

Darwin C (1998) The expression of the emotions in man and animals (3rd ed.). New York: Oxford University Press.

Davis M (1997) Neurobiology of fear responses: The role of the amygdala. J Neuropsychiatry Clin Neurosic, 9:382–402.

Fonagy P & Steele H (1991) Maternal representations of attachment during pregnancy predict the organization of infant–mother attachment at one year of age. Child Dev, 62:880–893.

Francis D, Diorio J, LaPlante P, Weaver S, Seckl JR, & Meaney MJ (1996) The role of early environmental events in regulating neuroendocrine development: Moms, pups, stress, and glucocorticoid receptors. *Ann of NY Acad Sci*, 794:136–52.

Freud S (1959) Inhibitions, symptoms, and anxiety. In J Strachey (Ed.), *Standard edition of the complete psychological works of Sigmund Freud* (Vol. 20, pp. 87–174). London: Hogarth Press.

Freud S (1962) The neuro-psychoses of defense. In J Strachey (Ed.), *Standard edition of the complete psychological works of Sigmund Freud* (Vol. 2, pp. 45–61). London: Hogarth Press.

Furmark T, Fischer H, Wik G, Larsson M, & Fredrikson M (1997) The amygdala and individual differences in human fear conditioning. *NeuroReport*, 8:3957–3960.

Gilbert P (2001) Evolution and social anxiety: The role of attraction, social competition, and social hierarchies. *Psychiatric Clin North Am*, 24:723–751.

Goddard AW & Charney DS (1997) Toward an integrated neurobiology of panic disorder. *J Clin Psychiatry*, 58:4–11.

Goldstein RB, Weissman MM, Adams PB, Horwath E, Lish JD, Charney D, Woods SW, Sobin C, & Wickramaratne PJ (1994) Psychiatric disorders in relatives of probands with panic disorder and/or major depression. *Arch Gen Psychiatry*, 51:383–394.

Graeff FG (1997) Serotonergic systems. *Psychiatr Clin North Am*, 20:723–739.

Graeff FG, Viana MB, & Mora PO (1997) Dual role of 5-HT in defense and anxiety. *Neurosci Biobehav Rev*, 21:791–799.

Graham P & Rutter M (1973) Psychiatric disorder in the young adolescent: A follow-up study. *Proc R So Med*, 66:1226–1229.

Gray JA & McNaughton N (1996) The neuropsychology of anxiety: Reprise. In DA Hope (Ed.), *Perspectives on anxiety, panic, and fear* (Vol. 43, pp. 61–134). Nebraska Symposium on Motivation. Omaha: University of Nebraska Press.

Harlow HF, Plubell PE, & Baysinger CM (1973) Induction of psychological death in rhesus monkeys. *J Autism Child Schizophr*, 3:299–307.

Ialongo N, Edelsohn G, Werthamer–Larsson L, Crockett L, & Kellam S (1996) The course of aggression in first-grade children with and without comorbid anxious symptoms. *J Abnorm Child Psychol*, 24:445–456.

Insel TR (1977) A neurobiological basis of social attachment. *Am J Psychiatry*, 154:726–735.

Kagan J (1997) Temperament and the reactions to unfamiliarity. *Child Dev*, 68:139–143.

Kagan J, Reznick JS, & Snidman N (1988) Biological bases of childhood shyness. *Science*, 240:167–171.

Kalin NH (1993) The neurobiology of fear. *Sci Am*, 268:94–101.

Kerr M, Tremblay RE, Pagani L, & Vitaro F (1997) Boys' behavioral inhibition and the risk of later delinquency. *Arch Gen Psychiatry*, 54:809–816.

Klein DF (1993) False suffication alarms, spontaneous panics, and related conditions: An integrative hypothesis. *Arch Gen Psychiatry*, 50:306–317.

Klein RG (1995) Anxiety disorders. In M Rutter, E Taylor, & L Hersov (Eds.), *Child and adolescent psychiatry: Modern approaches* (3rd ed., pp. 351–374). London: Blackwell Scientific.

LaBar KS, Gatenby JC, Gore JC, LeDoux JE, & Phelps EA (1998) Human amygdala activation during conditioned fear acquisition and extinction: A mixed-trial fMRI study. *Neuron*, 20:937–945.

Lapouse RL & Monk MA (1958) An epidemiological study of behavior characteristics in children. *Am J Public Health*, 48:1134–1144.

LeDoux J (1996) *The emotional brain: The mysterious underpinnings of emotional life*. New York: Simon & Schuster.

Liu D, Diorio J, Tannenbaum B, Caldji C, Francis D, Freedman A, Sharma S, Pearson D, Plotsky PM, & Meaney MJ (1997) Maternal care, hippocampal glucocorticoid receptors, and hypothalamic–pituitary–adrenal responses to stress. *Science*, 277:1659–1662.

Marks IM (1987) *Fears, phobias, and rituals: Panic, anxiety, and their disorders*. New York: Oxford University Press.

McGuire M & Troisi A (1998) *Darwinian psychiatry*. New York: Oxford University Press.

McNish KA, Gewirtz JC, & Davis M (1997) Evidence of contextual fear after lesions of the hippocampus: A disruption freezing but not fear-potentiated startle. *J Neurosci*, 17:9353–9360.

Meaney MJ, Bhatnagar S, Diorio J, Larocque S, Francis D, O'Donnell O, Shanks N, Sharma S, Smythe J, & Viau V (1993) Molecular basis for the development of individual differences in the hypothalamic–pituitary–adrenal stress response. *Cell Mol Neurobiol*, 13:321–347.

Mitchell S & Rosa P (1981) Boyhood behavior problems as precursors of criminality: A fifteen year follow-up study. *J Child Psychol Psychiatry*, 22:19–33.

Moffitt TE (1993) Adolescence-limited and life-course-persistent antisocial behavior: A developmental taxonomy. *Psychol Rev*, 100:674–701.

Nesse RM (1999) Proximate and evolutionary studies of anxiety, stress and depression: Synergy at the interface. *Neurosci Biobehav Rev*, 23:895–903.

Neese RM & Williams GC (1994) *Why we get sick*. New York: Random House.

Ohman A (1986) Face the beast and fear the face: Animal and social fears as prototypes for evolutionary analyses of emotion. *Psychophysiology*, 23:123–145.

Panksepp J (1998) *Affective neuroscience: The foundations of human and animal emotions*. New York: Oxford University Press.

Panksepp J, Newman JD, & Insel TR (1992) Critical conceptual issues in the analysis of separation-distress systems of the brain. In KT Strongman (Ed.), *International review of studies on emotion* (Vol. 2, pp. 51–71). New York: Wiley.

Papp LA, Klein DF, Gorman JM, Martinez JM, Coplan JD, Normal RG, Cole R, de Jesus MJ, Ross D, & Goetz R (1997) Respiratory psychophysiology of panic disorder: Three respiratory challenges in 98 subjects. *Am J Psychiatry*, 154:1557–1565.

Peterson BS & Klein JE (1997) Neuroimaging of Tourette's syndrome neurobiological substrate. *Child Adolesc Psychiatr Clin North Am*, 6:343–364.

Pine DS (1997) Childhood anxiety disorders. *Curr Opin Ped*, 9:329–338.

Pine DS, Cohen E, Cohen P, & Brook JS (2000) Social phobia and the persistence of conduct problems. *J Child Psychol Psychiatry*, 41(5):651–665.

Pine DS, Cohen P, Gurley D, Brook J, & Ma Y (1998a) The risk for early adulthood anxiety and depressive disorders in adolescents with anxiety and depressive disorders. *Arch Gen Psychiatry*, 55:56–64.

Pine DS, Coplan J, Klein R, Papp L, Hoven C, Martinez J, Moreau D, Klein D, & Gorman J (1997) CO_2 hypersensitivity in children and adolescents with anxiety disorders. *Proc Am Acad Child and Adolesc Psychiatry* (Abstract, NR-32).

Pine DS, Coplan JD, Papp LA, Klein RG, Martinez JM, Kovalenko P, Tancer N, Moreau D, Dummit ES, Shaffer D, Klein DF, & Gorman JM (1998b) Ventilatory physiology in children and adolescents with anxiety disorders. *Arch Gen Psychiatry*, 55:123–129.

Pine DS, Grun J, & Gorman JM (1998c) Anxiety disorders. In SJ Enna & JT Coyle (Eds.), *Pharmacological management of neurological and psychiatric disorders* (pp. 53–94). New York: McGraw-Hill.

Raine A (1993) *The psychopathology of crime: Criminal behavior as a clinical disorder.* San Diego, CA: Academic Press.

Raine A, Reynolds C, Venables PH, Mednick SA, & Farrington DP (1998) Fearlessness, stimulation-seeking, and large body size at age 3 years as early predispositions to childhood aggression at age 11 years. *Arch Gen Psychiatry*, 55:745–51.

Rauch SL, Savage CR, Alpert NM, Fischman AJ, & Jenike MA (1997) The functional neuroanatomy of anxiety: A study of three disorders using positron emission tomography and symptom provocation. *Biol Psychiatry*, 42:446–452.

Rosen JB & Schulkin J (1998) From normal fear to pathological anxiety. *Psychol Rev*, 105:325–350.

Sapolsky RM (1992) *Stress, the aging brain, and the mechanisms of neuron death.* Cambridge, MA: MIT Press.

Sapolsky R (2000). Glucocorticoids and hippocampal atrophy in neuropsychiatric disorders. *Arch Gen Psychiatry* 57:925–934.

Sapolsky RM (2004) Is impaired neurogenesis relevant to the affective symptoms of depression? *Biol Psychiatry*, 56:137–139.

Schneier FR, Johnson J, Hornig CD, Liebowitz MR, & Weissman MM (1992) Social phobia. Comorbidity and morbidity in an epidemiologic sample. *Arch Gen Psychiatry*, 49:282–288.

Schneirla TC & Rosenblatt JD (1961) Behavioral organization and genesis of the social bond in insects and mammals. *Am J Ortho*, 31:223–253.

Shapiro T & Jegede RO (1973) School phobia, a babel of tongues. *J Autism Child Schizophr*, 3:168–186.

Verhulst FC, van der Ende J, Ferdinand RF, & Kasius MC (1997) The prevalence of DSM-III-R diagnoses in a national sample of Dutch adolescents. *Arch Gen Psychiatry*, 54:329–336.

Walker DL & Davis M (1997) Double dissociation between the involvement of the bed nucleus of the stria terminalis and the central nucleus of the amygdala in startle increases produced by conditioned versus unconditioned fear. *J Neurosci*, 17:9375–9383.

Warren SL, Huston L, Egeland B, & Sroufe LA (1997) Child and adolescent anxiety disorders and early attachment. *J Am Acad Child Adolesc Psychiatry*, 36:637–644.

Whalen PJ, Rauch SL, Etcoff NL, McInerney SC, Lee MB, & Jenike MA (1998) Masked presentation of emotional facial expressions modulate amygdala activity without explicit knowledge. *J Neurosci*, 18:411–418.

CHAPTER 5

An Evolutionary Perspective on Childhood Depression

CYNTHIA R. PFEFFER

Empirically tested observations of children and adolescents suggest that depression is a heterogeneous phenomenon that can exist with varying intensity and other characteristics (Compas et al., 1993). Specifically, depression occurs as a symptom of sadness for an unspecified time. It occurs as a syndrome or constellation of emotions and behaviors that occur together in an identifiable pattern at a rate that exceeds chance. It occurs as a disorder that includes a cluster of symptoms that characteristically co-occur and are associated with significant levels of discomfort and impairment.

Sadness, the most common of these phenomena, is experienced in everyday life and is associated with life events, especially losses, but a depressive disorder is less prevalent. Some contend that depressive states represent an evolutionary phenomenon that is "a psychobiological response pattern" (Price et al., 1994, pp. 309) functioning as a conservation phenomenon to protect individuals from sequelae of adverse situations (Nesse, 2000; Gardner, 2001; Watson & Andrews, 2002; Nettle, 2004). This chapter expands a discussion of this concept and proposes that an understanding of childhood depression as an evolutionary phenomenon can promote the development of new diagnostic and treatment options and of research to improve the lives of children afflicted with or at risk for depression.

PROXIMATE CHARACTERIZATIONS
OF DEPRESSION

We experienced a time during the mid-1950s to the 1970s when it was thought that prepubertal depression did not exist (Rie, 1966) and that what was observed were depressive equivalents (Cytryn & McKnew, 1974; Malmquist, 1977). We are now convinced, largely through the initial empirical research of Puig-Antich (1987), that children of various ages do fit adult criteria for major depression and that prepubertal depressions have a chronic course and appear to be continuous with adolescent and adult depression (Kovacs et al., 1984a, 1984b, 1988).

Historical review of clinical observations and results of empirical psychosocial research highlight insights relating psychological etiological phenomena to depressive responses. For example, the psychoanalytic propositions of Freud (1957) discerned between sadness, as a mourning response to loss, and melancholia, a severe depressive sequel to a loss of one's internal mental representation of well-being. Freud proposed that melancholia is a state of intrapsychic dysfunction in which severe guilt is responsible for a protracted, intense mourning condition, which is evident as self-criticism, self-rejection, and internally directed anger. Others expanded these concepts by suggesting that not only may there be an objective loss, but that there is also an intrapsychic loss, that is, there is a basic loss of ego functioning, which leads to the basic affect of depression (Sandler & Joffe, 1965). The resultant manifestations are sensitivity to repeated disappointment, aggression toward the self, intense need for narcissistic gratification, loss of self-esteem, and feelings of helplessness. Spitz (1946), utilizing psychoanalytic principles and direct observations, reported on the entity of anaclitic depression, a preobjectal depressive state of infants who lack consistent caretaking and have not been able to build a stable representation of a caretaker.

Cognitive features of depression, including a triad of negative views of oneself, of the world, and of the future, are important in evaluating one's experiences, interpersonal activities, mood, motivation, and behavior (Beck, 1987; Kazdin, 1990). Learned helplessness, another feature of depression, is manifest by social impairment, passivity, and change in psychomotor activity (Seligman, 1975). Deficits in social skills and problem-solving methods have been related to depression (D'Zurilla & Nezu, 1982; Kazdin, 1990). Lewinsohn (1974) proposed depression to be a result of loss or reduction of reinforcement provided by the environment for acquisition of skills and understanding of consequences to environmental events. A child, therefore, may become passive and withdrawn and exhibit other symptoms of depression. This is illustrated by observing the consequences for young children who are raised by depressed mothers who are less rewarding to their children, promote more conflict in the family, and may be more detached from their children. This maternal behavior promotes in children feelings of resentment, anger, depression, and other features of dysfunction.

This historical review suggests new considerations about sadness and depressive affects. Such affects may serve adaptive functions that can carry children and adolescents through the developmental cycle into adulthood (Nettle, 2004). However, it is also evident that extremes of affect can be lethal and that if the homeostatic balance is overextended into a depressive disorder, the developmental process is impeded and the expression of chronic depression leads to poor socialization manifested as alienation or maladaptive roles.

EXAMPLES OF CHILDHOOD DEPRESSION

The following examples describe the characteristic symptoms of depression, features of comorbid psychopathology, and environmental factors operative in augmenting the children's level of distress. They highlight varied presentations of the adaptive and psychopathological features of depression.

Child 1

A 10-year-old boy with a history of physical abuse in infancy was hospitalized in a psychiatric facility after running away from a residential treatment center. He wanted to kill himself by jumping off a nearby bridge. He was found wandering on a country road by the police, who brought him to a hospital emergency room.

Three months before this episode of suicidal threat, the child entered the residential treatment center because he was unmanageable, irritable, and angry at home. His father, a harsh disciplinarian, believed that his son was possessed by the devil and deserved to be punished for his unwillingness to cooperate with family life. The child's mother was distraught by the conflict between her son and her husband. She was unable to help them resolve their intense animosity. In recent months, the child had withdrawn from the family and was truant from school.

During the emergency service intake interview, the child appeared depressed. He held his head down and spoke slowly without detail. At times, he was tearful. He stated that he felt hopeless. He wanted to die because he felt he had no place in this world. He thought that whatever he did was viewed by his father as insufficient and bad. He reported that while he lived at the residential treatment center, he was disliked and threatened by his peers because he would not agree to do what they wanted. He was preoccupied with feelings of rejection by his family. He described difficulty in falling asleep and having nightmares each night. He was in a state of despair and could not concentrate on schoolwork.

This child was diagnosed as having a major depressive disorder with suicidal ideation and a comorbid oppositional-defiant disorder (ODD). Because his symptoms of depression were chronic, he was also diagnosed as having a dysthymic disorder. His family life, school activities, and peer relationships were impaired. This child had lived with long-standing family adversity. He experienced a chronic state of despair and helplessness about not being able to change his situation. Withdrawal served to protect him from problematic interactions at home and in school. Anger, irritability, and oppositional behavior were associated with his efforts to challenge his father's strict family rules. However, because he felt extremely helpless and hopeless, he wished to die. His runaway episode and suicidal ideation signaled his need for more intensive intervention. Evaluation of these extreme symptoms stimulated his admission to a child psychiatric hospital unit where treatment could decrease his impairing condition and ameliorate the intensity of the family dysfunction.

Child 2

A 14-year-old girl told her school guidance counselor that she planned to kill herself by taking her mother's antidepressant medication. She wished to die because a boy she liked had begun to date her best friend. The girl reported being angry at her mother because her mother would not allow her to date this boy. She stated that her mother only wanted her to do household chores. In addition, she stated that her mother wanted her to be home after school so that she could complete her homework and get high grades. The girl described how her mother often withdrew from the family, seldom wanted to take her daughter anywhere, and stated that every family member must help maintain the routines at home. Her parents had divorced 3 years before this suicidal episode. The girl saw her father every other weekend when he was home. She was upset that since he began his new job, he was away often and could not be with her. This increased her loneliness and helplessness.

This child suffered from chronic feelings of depression, helplessness, isolation, and poor concentration. She tried to endure a problematic family situation with an absent father and an intolerant, unempathic mother. The fact that her mother had a serious mood disorder increased this adolescent's risk for a mood disorder. The girl's wishes to have a boyfriend were developmentally appropriate. The thwarting of these desires and the loss of support from her father increased her despair. She felt she had to tolerate her situation and could not change it. Because of increased sadness and despair, she withdrew from family interactions and was intensely preoccupied with wishing to have a boyfriend.

DOES DEPRESSED MOOD HAVE AN EVOLUTIONARY ADVANTAGE?

To understand the question raised, it is necessary to consider a basic evolutionary premise of whether depression confers an adaptive advantage that ultimately enhances fitness, thereby ensuring the reproductive potential necessary for the survival of a species. Specifically, it can be hypothesized that depression is a set of biologically based adaptive mechanisms that are invoked in response to changes in social structure. These adaptive mechanisms function to protect against the loss of necessary resources such as family, friends, possessions, social status, education, and so forth (Nesse & Williams, 1994). Although depression could have an evolutionary function in aiding people to cope with unpropitious situations (Nesse, 2000), it may also be possible that depression per se is not adaptive, but rather that some of the traits and characteristics associated with proclivities for depression are (Nettle, 2004).

Elucidation of evolutionary principles related to depression requires one to have knowledge about the primordial social structure and communication patterns of humans and to relate these to what has been discovered about similar reaction patterns in other species. An important feature of the social structure of humans is that children have a period of intense attachment to a caretaking adult, a mechanism of survival that protects the young from environmental adversities during rapid periods of development. It is hypothesized that the capacity to form such an intense attachment is phylogenetically determined and is evident across species (Bowlby, 1982). During this early attachment period, extensive brain maturation occurs and social skills are acquired. It has been observed that symptoms of depression involving sadness and changes in appetite, sleep, activity, and immunity are characteristic of children who have lost a parent or are raised by mothers who are unable to provide consistent parenting (Bowlby, 1982). Such depressed children exhibit social withdrawal, which may be hypothesized to "foster an avoidance of an aversive state of dysregulation associated with insensitive or unresponsive parenting" (Cummings & Davies, 1994, p. 78). Thus, sadness and associated features of cognitive constriction and motor retardation after loss of parental resources may reduce a child's tendencies to overestimate personal capacities and the security of circumstances and to ready a child to disengage from a hopeless situation and to consider implementing new social relationships (Bowlby, 1982; Nesse, 2000; Nesse & Williams, 1994). Aberrations in mother–child attachment may sensitize the child to future inconsistencies in interpersonal relations (Bowlby, 1982). Such sensitization, an adaptive mechanism, may be expressed as depression, which enables a process of reassessment of current circumstances and readjustment of social bonds.

Price and colleagues (1994) focused on another feature of social structure in proposing an evolutionary hypothesis that depression is an adaptive mechanism for yielding in competitive situations. They noted that depression is an "involuntary subordinate strategy" that (1) prevents an individual from continuing a lost competition by inhibiting aggressive behavior to rivals and experiencing a subjective sense of incapacity; (2) signals defeat and inability to resume the competition; and (3) enables an acceptance of capitulation, which leads to reconciliation and termination of conflict. This hypothesis suggests that depression mediates social processes regarding social hierarchy, which is an elemental feature of the preservation of the human species. Coping mechanisms to satisfactorily negotiate the human hierarchical social schema develop early in life and are related to the qualities of the parent–child relationship.

Social hierarchical schemas in humans and other species regulate the transfer of power and breeding opportunities (Price et al., 1994). Depression ensures that the loser yields and thereby survives. Self-esteem is a basic element of the mechanisms of competitive behavior. Those with high self-esteem tend to exhibit highly competitive strategies, and those with low self-esteem have a reconciliatory or de-escalation strategy. The low self-esteem strategy is a form of altruistic behavior. It is notable that this hypothesis of social competition is related to sexual selection and in humans, as in other species, involves a phylogenetic mechanism for creating social asymmetry between previously equal adults (Price et al., 1994).

Theories of socialization processes suggest that the actions of socialization agents, such as parents and teachers, are instrumental in the development of coping strategies in humans, especially those that are gender-specific. As a result of socializing processes, girls show higher levels of self-evaluative concerns, such as lower expectations for future success, more maladaptive causal attributions for future successful outcomes, and negative behavioral and evaluative reactions to failure (Ruble et al., 1993). These characteristic modes of coping with interpersonal stress are suggested to be important in risk for depression. Nolen-Hoeksema and Girgus (1994) suggested that gender differences in rates of depression in adolescence were related to trends in which females, as compared with males, are more likely to be lower on aggression and dominance in interpersonal circumstances before adolescence, but that these factors interact with psychosocial challenges in adolescence to increase risk for depression. Notably, adequately designed systematic studies regarding pubertal and other physiological factors related to brain maturation and differences in regional activation of the brain are needed to identify relations that are important in understanding gender differences in rates of depression in adolescents. Although such studies are relatively rare, some suggest that biological-developmental factors account for only a small proportion of the variance in gender differences in rates of depression among male and female adolescents (Angold & Worthman, 1993).

NEUROPHYSIOLOGICAL FEATURES
RELATED TO DEPRESSION

The capacity for brain plasticity, especially in critical phases of development, endows a child with adaptive mechanisms utilizable in circumstances in which loss of resources has occurred. Theories of social information processing provide a neurophysiological basis of understanding how early socialization processes exert strong influences on brain plasticity at critical periods of development that eventuate in differential rates of depression at various developmental stages.

Such theories propose that a person's behavior as a response to a situational stimulus is a function of a sequence of processes in discrete neurophysiological pathways that involve (1) encoding of relevant aspects of the stimulus; (2) mental representation by which meaning is applied to the encoded stimulus; (3) response accessing in which the mental representation evokes behavioral and affective responses; (4) response evaluation that involves a decision-making process; and (5) enactment in which the selected response is transformed into behavior (Dodge, 1993). It has been postulated that "for all social mammals there are distinctive neuropsychological organismic states that underlie behavior patterns correlated with social position" (Gardner, 1982). Depression may be defined in terms of neurophysiological processing that involves helpless attributions and hopeless expectations, especially in response to loss of attachments or failure.

Post (1992) described another feature of brain plasticity in his hypothesis of neurobiological mechanisms for depression that linked psychosocial stress at critical periods with induction of the proto-oncogene c-fos and related gene transcription factors. Post (1992) suggested that depressive episodes are mediated by the stimulation of gene expression. Memory traces of stress and resultant neurobiological responses, especially at critical periods, become permanent and affect subsequent neurophysiological responses of neurotransmitters, neuroreceptors, neuropeptides, intracellular functions of second messengers, and so on, to stress. Post further noted that a first episode of a mood disorder is more likely to be associated with more severe psychosocial stress than a subsequent episode. This genetic-sensitization hypothesis highlights that the functioning of regulatory genes may change in response to stress and that the course of mood disorders may progress with manifestations of symptoms whose onset and offset for specific, recurrent episodes may occur out of context of significant psychosocial stress. Post noted that specific types of psychosocial stress receive specific neurophysiological responses in distinct neuronal pathways. Thus, such a genetic-stimulation hypothesis may be studied in regard to specific contextual stimuli, such as loss of social resources or social hierarchy, and the social information processing related to depression.

Accumulating results from research in humans point out the important role of an imbalance of the adrenal–corticosteroid system as a neurophysiological response agent to stress and a correlate of depression (Dubrovsky, 1993). The activity of this system is heightened during time of stress. The hypothalamic–pituitary–adrenocortical axis functions to mobilize energy needed to cope with a stressful situation. Such responses are mediated by genetic processes that account for interindividual vulnerability to depression. Adrenal–corticosteroids exert trophic effects on the dentate gyrus of the hippocampus, a site in the limbic region of the brain that has influence on multiple features that characterize depression, such as mood, memory, attention, and activity (Dubrovsky, 1993). Abnormalities in the balance of adrenal–corticosteroid, especially at critical periods (see, e.g., Amiel-Tison et al., 2004), may alter hippocampal functioning with resultant aberrations in encoding of events as memories, which may manifest as cognitive distortions that are frequently observable in depression. Furthermore, serotonin and norepinephrine stimulate release of corticotropin-releasing factor, which affects release of adrenocorticotropic hormone (ACTH) and adrenocorticosteroid. Thus, altered serotonergic function may initiate a cascade of responses that impact on adrenocorticosteroid actions on hippocampal formation, which may influence cognitive and other features of depression (Sapolsky, 2000, 2004). These neurobiological responses that are related to depression are stimulated by the impact of environmental events, especially at critical developmental periods, with long-term effects on physical and mental health, including propensities to develop depression (Amiel-Tison et al., 2004; Meaney, 2001).

These studies suggest important issues in understanding the evolutionary features of brain plasticity and their relations to childhood depression. Specifically, basic neuroregulatory genes appear to be associated with symptoms of depression, and their functioning may be altered in response to environmental stimuli. However, if stimulated in excess, their neuroregulatory functioning may be become dysregulated in relation to external stimuli, thereby affecting the course of depression.

STUDIES OF NONHUMAN SPECIES

Comparative studies of species are an aid in understanding evolutionary mechanisms that maintain survival capabilities of an organism. Studies of nonhuman primates, species that have similar genetic background to humans, are valuable for augmenting knowledge about socialization processes and neurobiological indices relevant to depression in humans.

Higley and Suomi (1996) described their extensive observational studies of socialization in rhesus macaques. They noted that the main types of stressors of such primates involve loss of a loved one, change in social relationships, and interpersonal conflicts. They emphasized that some behaviors, such as withdrawal, appear to be similar to depression in humans and enable an individual to cope with such stresses and to seek new social situations. These responses are controlled by the central nervous system, whose development, in turn, is influenced by early experiences. As rhesus macaques mature, they must learn to cope with adversity by seeking social support to maintain their resources. Developmental distinctions in behavior are prominent, such that in late childhood and early adolescence social roles and coping methods of male and female rhesus macaques become dissimilar. Each gender must integrate into the adult social dominance hierarchy. These observations are important in supporting hypotheses about humans regarding gender role differences and social-competition processes. Their studies suggest that neurobiological indices, such as concentrations of serotonin and its metabolite 5-hydroxyindoleacetic acid, are correlated positively with social competence and social dominance rankings in rhesus macaques, thereby suggesting issues that may be pertinent in understanding neurobiological adaptations that are related to manifestations of depression in humans.

Rosenblum and Paully (1987), studying nonhuman primates, emphasized that, in addition to genetic propensities, early environmental experiences, such as social separation, impact on the development of neural systems related to expression of depression. Notably, the social context of rearing influences the nature of parent–child attachment and responses to social separation. For example, pigtail macaques living in their natural habitat form less cohesive groups. These individuals tend to live in isolation. Infants are guarded closely by their mothers until weaning, which occurs aggressively when the time of rebreeding approaches. In comparison, bonnet macaques live in cohesive, gregarious groups with close contact between individuals. Grooming, touching, and sharing of infant care occur readily among group members, and weaning is a gradual, nonpunitive process. Studies of these of macaques indicate that these different weaning experiences are associated with future types of responses to loss. For example, pigtail macaques experience severe depressive reactions following social loss, whereas bonnet macaques rarely exhibit depressive symptoms at times of loss.

Experimental studies provide additional evidence that environmental influences on the parenting of infants affect the security of infants and that such interactions affect long-term sequelae of the infants (Rosenblum & Paully, 1987). Specifically, bonnet macaque mothers, when placed in environments that require them to forage for food, in comparison with control bonnet mothers that are provided with ample amounts of food, have infants that appear to be more independent of the mothers. However, such infants, as compared with infants whose mothers were away from them less often and for less time, exhibited more overt hostility and less affiliative behavior. These infants of mothers that were required to forage for food were observed to have severe depressive symptoms and were more subordinate and less able to learn competent coping skills necessary for the environment. Thus, the reaction to loss in nonhuman primates is not fixed but influenced by genetic factors, individual characteristics, and environmental influences.

Neuroendocrine effects have also been identified as heightened hypothalamic–pituitary–adrenocortical axis responses to acute separation. Prospective research utilizing randomly assigned nonhuman primate subjects suggested that there were significant effects of early environments on susceptibility for adult mood and anxiety disorders and that these effects were associated with neurodevelopmental alterations of noradrenergic and serotonergic systems (Rosenblum et al., 1994).

Other pioneering studies of rodents (Meaney et al., 1996a, 1996b) and nonhuman primates (Coplan et al., 1996) suggested that the development of the hypothalamic–pituitary–adrenocortical (HPA) axis response to stressful stimuli is altered by early environmental events. Specifically, animals exposed to short periods of infant stimulation exhibit decreased HPA responsivity to stress, but maternal separation, physical trauma, and endotoxin exposure enhance HPA responsivity to stress—effects that persist over the lifetime (Meaney et al., 1996a). These studies suggest that early environmental events can influence the development of stable individual differences to stress responses. It can be inferred that such effects on the HPA axis may enhance vulnerability to pathological coping with environmental stressful situations and serve as a potential model for understanding the relationship between HPA dysregulation and depression in humans.

RATIONALE FOR A PARADIGM SHIFT FOR CHILDHOOD DEPRESSION

In general, theories of depression have focused on proximate features of etiology such as actual or perceived loss and proximate characteristics involving cognitive styles and skills. Rarely have such theories considered the adaptive features of depression as a function of a basic neurophysiological design for the survival of the human species. Current diagnostic considerations utilizing DSM classification of depression involve an atheoretical phenomenological classification that emphasizes signs and symptoms as diagnostic criteria that, when clustered together, represent a psychiatric disorder. The fact that prevalence of mood disorders is low (Fleming & Offord, 1990) and that they are usually diagnosed to be comorbid with other disorders, such as anxiety disorders, raises issues about the specificity of current diagnostic methods and the need for a paradigm shift away from proximate characterization of etiological stresses to that of ultimate cause, such as offered by an evolutionary explanation. It is possible that natural selection has linked several negative moods to adapt to different kinds of unpropitious situations and that brain mechanisms that mediate these responses are interrelated (Nesse, 2000).

An evolutionary explanation emphasizes why some individuals may exhibit depression. It suggests that all humans have a basic neurobiological propensity to manifest depression under certain external circumstances, such as when necessary resources are depleted. It offers the potential to distinguish between this basic propensity, as an adaptive mechanism, and a dysregulation of this propensity that may be manifest as an abnormality or an illness. Such an approach suggests that the context in which children exhibit depression must be evaluated. For example, a child's sadness may be an adaptive mechanism that signals a "cry for help" in situations when the child lacks sufficient social network support, such as after parental separation/divorce, parental death, or a child's transfer to a new foster home. A cognitive attribution of despair may enable a child to give up hope that restitution of the loss is possible and to think about establishing new relationships. Vegetative symptoms of appetite, sleep, and motor changes may enable a child to conserve resources and retreat from lost competitive situations.

Evidence for the importance of environmental influences, such as the qualities of the social structure and changes in social relations, on the prevalence of depression has been presented by research suggesting that although genetic factors are related to the etiology of depressive symptoms and to individual differences in severity of depressive symptoms, common environmental factors are significantly more associated with extreme levels of depressive symptoms than heritability (Eley, 1997; Rende et al., 1993).

Further support for an environmental influence on prevalence of depression has been obtained from research suggesting that there is an increase in depression in adolescent cohorts born after World War II and that a genetic etiology is unlikely (Klerman et al., 1985). More plausible explanations may reflect the effects of extensive environmental changes, such as significant social changes related to increased mobility, competition for resources, and family dissolution. It can be postulated that the increased prevalence of depression may be a manifestation of a basic adaptive propensity to conserve or restore actual or perceived scarce resources. This example highlights the importance of considering a paradigm shift toward an evolutionary explanation highlighting the adaptive aspects of depression that involve the relations between neurobiological plasticity, developmentally sensitive periods, and contextual factors (Allen & Badcock, 2003).

FUTURE DIRECTIONS FOR CONSIDERING THE RELATION OF DEPRESSION AND ADAPTIVE PROCESSES

This chapter suggests that a paradigm shift is needed that applies knowledge of evolutionary principles to the diagnosis, treatment, and research of childhood depression. Evolutionary principles suggest that depressive symptoms may be part of a basic inborn phylogenetic mechanism that has evolutionary value in the schemas of the social communication and social structural patterns of humans. Genetic mechanisms responsive to specific stimuli regarding change of social circumstances, such as loss of resources and social hierarchy, may activate various neurochemical processes that are associated with the onset of depressive symptoms. Social-information processing, with its neurophysiological underpinnings, may be responsible for molding the patterns that are inherent in depressive disorders. In the extreme, mood disorders occur and have been shown to be most prevalent among families with a strong intergenerational history of mood disorders. Thus, genetic vulnerability may be associated with a hypersensitive baseline condition that, when interacting with specific psychosocial stress—for example, that related to social changes involving loss of resources—may precipitate the extreme symptomatology evident as mood disorders. New venues for diagnosing, treating, and preventing depressive disorders may be benefited by considering these concepts.

The effect on socialization experiences at critically sensitive periods to the development of social attributions is a potentially important arena for new research. Empirical investigations focusing on the impact of social forces on development may enable the design of preventive interventions that are likely to reduce the prevalence of mood disorders. For example, early childhood developmental factors may be influenced by designing methods of promoting effective parenting skills, fostering consistent attachment bonds between mother and child, and identifying social attributions that influence gender-specific role differences. Research relating genetic vulnerability and contextual experiences, especially at critical time periods, is essential to identify individuals who may be at risk for pathological states of depression. Research may elucidate treatment paradigms that may supersede current approaches of targeting symptoms and focus on promoting adaptive mechanisms involving cognitive appraisal of circumstances and modification of situational conditions.

REFERENCES

Allen NB & Badcock PB (2003) The social risk hypothesis of depressed mood: Evolutionary, psychosocial, and neurobiological perspectives. *Psychol Bull*, 129(6):887–913.

Amiel-Tison C, Cabrol D, Denver R, Jarreau PH, Papiernik E, & Piazza PV (2004) Fetal adaptation to stress: Part II. Evolutionary aspects; stress-induced hippocampal damage; long-term effects on behavior; consequences on adult health. *Early Hum Dev*, 78:81–94.

Angold A & Worthman CW (1993) Puberty inset of gender differences in rates of depression: A developmental, epidemiologic and neuroendocrine perspective. *J Affective Disord*, 29:145–158.

Beck AT (1987) Cognitive models of depression. *J Cogn Psychother*, 1:5–37.

Bowlby J (1982) *Attachment and loss: Attachment.* New York: Basic Books.

Compas BE, Ey S, & Grant KE (1993) Taxonomy, assessment, and diagnosis of depression during adolescence. *Psychological Bull*, 114:323–344.

Coplan JD, Andrews MW, Rosenblum LA, Owens MJ, Friedman S, Gorman JM, & Nemeroff CB (1996) Persistent elevations of cerebrospinal fluid concentrations of corticotropin-releasing factor in adult nonhuman primates exposed to early-life stressors: Implications for the pathophysiology of mood and anxiety disorders. *Proc Nat Acad Sci*, 93:1619–1623.

Cummings EM & Davies PT (1994) Maternal depression and child development. *J Child Psychol Psychiatry*, 35:73–112.

Cytryn L & McKnew DH (1974) Factors influencing the changing clinical expression of the depressive processes in children. *Am J Psychiatry*, 131:879–881.

Dodge KA (1993) Social-cognitive mechanisms in the development of conduct disorder and depression. *Annu Rev Psychol*, 44:559–584.

Dubrovsky B (1993) Effects of adrenal cortex hormones on limbic structures: Some experimental and clinical correlations related to depression. *J Psychiatry Neurosci*, 18:4–16.

D'Zurilla TJ & Nezu A (1982) Social problem solving in adults. In PC Kendall (Ed.), *Advances in cognitive-behavioral research and therapy* (Vol. 1, pp. 202–274). New York: Academic Press.

Eley TC (1997) Depressive symptoms in children and adolescents: Etiological links between normality and abnormality: A research note. *J Child Psychol Psychiatry*, 38:861–865.

Fleming JE & Offord DR (1990) Epidemiology of childhood depressive disorders: A critical review. *J Am Acad Child Adolesc Psychiatry*, 29:571–580.

Freud S (1957) Mourning and melancholia. In J Strachey (Ed.), *Standard edition of the complete psychological works of Sigmund Freud* (Vol. 14, pp. 243–258). London: Hogarth Press.

Gardner R (1982) Mechanisms in manic–depressive disorder: An evolutionary model. *Arch Gen Psychiatry*, 39:1436–1441.

Gardner R (2001). Evolutionary perspectives on stress and affective disorder. *Semin Clin Neuropsychiatry*, 6:32–42.

Higley JD & Suomi SJ (1996) Reactivity and social competence affect individual differences to severe stress in children: Investigations using nonhuman primates. In CR Pfeffer (Ed.), *Severe stress and mental disturbance in children* (pp. 3–58). Washington, DC: American Psychiatric Press.

Kazdin AE (1990) Childhood depression. *J Child Psychol Psychiatry*, 31:121–160.

Kendler KS (1996) Parenting: A genetic-epidemiologic perspective. *Am J Psychiatry*, 153:11–20.

Klerman GL, Lavori PW, Rice J, Reich T, Endicott J, Andreasen NC, Keller MB, & Hirschfield RM (1985) Birth cohort trends in rates of major depressive disorder among relatives of patients with affective disorder. *Arch Gen Psychiatry*, 42:689–695.

Kovacs M, Feinberg TL, Crouse-Novak MA, Paulauskas SL, & Finkelstein R (1984a) Depressive disorders in childhood: I. A longitudinal perspective study of characteristics and recovery. *Arch Gen Psychiatry*, 41:229–237.

Kovacs M, Feinberg TL, Crouse-Novak MA, Paulauskas SL, Pollock M, & Finkelstein R (1984b) Depressive disorders in childhood: II. A longitudinal study of the risk for a subsequent major depression. *Arch Gen Psychiatry*, 41:643–649.

Kovacs M, Paulauskas S, Gatsonis C, & Richards C (1988) Depressive disorders in childhood: III. A longitudinal study of comorbidity with and risk for conduct disorders. *J Affective Disord*, 15:205–217.

Lewinsohn PM (1974) Clinical and theoretical aspects of depression. In KS Calhoun, HE Adams, & KM Mitchell (Eds.), *Innovative treatment methods of psychopathology* (pp. 63–120). New York: Wiley.

Malmquist CP (1977) Childhood depression: A clinical and behavioral perspective. In JG Schulterbrandt & A Raskin (Eds.), *Depression in children: Diagnosis, treatment and conceptual models* (pp. 35–59). New York: Raven Press.

Meaney MJ (2001) Maternal care, gene expression, and the transmission of individual differences in stress reactivity across generations. *Annu Rev Neurosci*, 24:1161–92.

Meaney MJ, Bhatnagar S, Laroque S, McCormick C, Shanks N, Sharma S,

Smythe J, Viau V, & Plotsky PM (1996a) Early environment and the development of individual differences in the hypothalamic–pituitary–adrenal stress response. In CR Pfeffer (Ed.), *Severe stress and mental disturbance in children* (pp. 85–130). Washington DC: American Psychiatric Press.

Meaney MJ, Diorio J, Francis D, Widdowson J, LaPlante P, Caldji C, Sharma S, Seckl JR, & Plotsky PM (1996b) Early environmental regulation of forebrain glucocorticoid receptor gene expression: Implications for adrenocortical responses to stress. *Dev Neurosci*, 18:49–72.

Nesse R (2000) Is depression an adaptation? *Arch Gen Psychiatry*, 57:14–20.

Nesse RM & Williams GC (1994) *Why we get sick*. New York: Times Board, Random House.

Nettle D (2004). Evolutionary origins of depression: A review and reformulation. *J Affective Disord*, 81:91–102.

Nolen-Hoeksema S & Girgus JS (1994) The emergence of gender differences in depression during adolescence. *Psychol Bull*, 115:424–443.

Post RM (1992) Transduction of psychosocial stress into the neurobiology of recurrent affective disorder. *Am J Psychiatry*, 149:999–1010.

Price J, Sloman I, Gardner R Jr., Gilbert P, & Rohde P (1994) The social competition hypothesis of depression. *Br J Psychiatry*, 164:309–315.

Puig-Antich J (1987) Affective disorders in children and adolescents: Diagnostic validity and psychobiology. In HY Meltzer (Ed.), *Psychopharmacology: The third generation of progress* (pp. 843–859). New York: Raven Press.

Rende RD, Plomin R, Reiss D, & Hetherington EM (1993) Genetic and environmental influences on depressive symptomatology in adolescence: Individual differences and extreme scores. *J Child Psychol Psychiatry*, 34:1387–1398.

Rie HE (1966) Depression in childhood: A survey of some pertinent contributions. *J Am Acad Child Psychiatry*, 5:653–685.

Rosenblum LA, Coplan JD, Friedman S, Bassoff T, Gorman JM, & Andrews MW (1994) Adverse early experiences affect noradrenergic and serotonergic functioning in adult primates. *Biol Psychiatry*, 35:221–227.

Rosenblum LA & Paully GS (1987) Primate models of separation-induced depression. *Psychiatric Clin North Am*, 10:437–447.

Ruble DN, Greulich F, Pomerantz EM, & Gochberg B (1993) The role of gender-related processes in the development of sex differences in self—evaluation and depression. *J Affect Disord*, 29:97–128.

Sandler J & Joffe WG (1965) Notes on childhood depression. *Int J Psychoanalysis*, 46:88–96.

Sapolsky R (2000). Glucocorticoids and hippocampal atrophy in neuropsychiatric disorders. *Arch Gen Psychiatry* 57:925–934.

Sapolsky RM (2004) Is impaired neurogenesis relevant to the affective symptoms of depression? *Biol Psychiatry*, 56:137–139.

Seligman MEP (1975) *Helplessness: On depression, development, and death.* San Francisco: Freeman Press.

Spitz R (1946) Anaclitic depression. *Psychoanal Study Child*, 2:313–342.

Watson PJ & Andrews PW (2002) Toward a revised evolutionary adaptationist analysis of depression: The social navigation hypothesis. *J Affective Dis*, 72:1–14.

CHAPTER 6

Application of Evolutionary Models to Attention-Deficit/ Hyperactivity Disorder

PETER S. JENSEN, DAVID A. MRAZEK, PENNY KNAPP,
LAWRENCE STEINBERG, CYNTHIA R. PFEFFER,
JOHN SCHOWALTER, *and* THEODORE SHAPIRO

This chapter addresses the question of how one form of childhood traits and behaviors often thought to be solely internal biological dysfunctions—attention-deficit/hyperactivity disorder (ADHD)—can be reframed as adaptive responses to environmental contexts. Examining this "disorder" in relation to evolutionary theories of psychology and biology, we explore the thesis that evolutionary perspectives can explain the presence of ADHD traits in *some* children. This model is not intended to be all-encompassing, does not preclude other explanatory factors (genetic abnormalities, neurotoxins, head injury), and may even interact with other such factors. Nonetheless, given the current estimated frequency of ADHD (3–5%) (Richters et al., 1995), it is unlikely that such a "disorder" could be as prevalent in the human species if not maintained within the species by selection forces that conveyed certain advantages to some ADHD characteristics or other associated traits.

ADHD is characterized as a classical triad of symptoms: inattention, hyperactivity, and impulsivity. Leaving aside the co-occurrence of all three symptoms, we suggest that each of these "symptoms" can be adaptive in some instances. If this hypothesis is correct, what adaptive problems might each of these traits serve to solve, either in ancestral or modern-day environments?

INCREASED MOTOR ACTIVITY (HYPERACTIVITY)

For an organism to adapt successfully, it must constantly explore the environment for threats and opportunities. From this perspective, increased motor behavior and hyperactivity may be useful (particularly in ancestral hunter–gatherer environments) to assist in effective foraging, spotting of new opportunities, anticipating dangers, and so forth. Furthermore, increased motor behavior (especially during juvenile years) may serve to "wire the brain" to the external environment in a way to fit the environment, as well as to stimulate development of muscle and motor skills. Is this in the service of exploratory behavior, serving to develop a reservoir of experiences upon which the animal later draws? If this hypothesis is correct, one would theorize that animals adapted to food-scarce environments would show high degrees of motor behavior, perhaps even in the young who are not yet responsible for foraging (a testable assumption, both within and across species).

Yet does the juvenile animal always show increased motor behavior, or only under conditions where such motoric activity subserves adaptation? Consistent with our thesis, increased exploratory motor behavior usually occurs only in the context of proximity to the caretaking animal (hence, presumed safety), and a frightened animal (or child) who is characteristically highly motorically active will suppress motor activity during periods of separation from caregivers, in times of danger, or during situations with a high degree of novel stimuli (Bowlby, 1973). These straightforward observations illustrate the simple yet elegant premises of adaptational theory—motor behavior is expressed when it subserves adaptation and survival, and is suppressed when it does not, given sufficient time for evolutionary and selection forces to encode the behavioral repertoire within the species' genome. Not surprisingly, then, empirical studies of animals suggest that activity level involving speed, proportion of time active, and foraging effort is associated with resource acquisition among varying species (Werner & Anholt, 1993) and that speed and time of activity are reduced in the presence of predators (Lima & Dill, 1990).

ATTENTIONAL PROCESSES (SCANNING AND RAPIDLY SHIFTING ATTENTION)

Vigilance is necessary to monitor dangers and threats. Overfocused attention could be quite maladaptive in high-threat or highly novel environments, yet could be a productive use of cognitive capacities to allow for future planning when environmental threats or novel stimuli are minimal. Thus, according to our conceptualization, animals that are preyed upon or are in environments with a high ratio of predators to prey are more likely to have increased scanning behaviors. If the scanning strategy is malleable and "wired" during early development to fit the local environment in an organism-specific manner, within a given species animals that are raised in low-threat environments will show fewer scanning behaviors. In contrast, animals raised in higher-threat and/or highly novel stimulus-rich environments (where scanning is adaptive, learned, and in part species-specific) should show high scanning levels, even when this is no longer necessary during later development. Thus, although there may be evolved, adaptive reasons for the behavioral potentials existing within the species' genome, the environment shapes the tendencies of particular organisms within that species to express responses such as increased scanning behaviors, that is, "inattention" to a single, repetitive stimulus. Moreover, definitions of *over-* versus *underattention* are sensible only when situated within a given context and for specific classes of stimuli (e.g., those requiring active vs. passive listening) (Shibagaki & Yamanaka, 1990).

IMPULSIVITY

How about "impulsivity"? For the purposes of our thesis, we define impulsivity as an organism's quick response to environmental cues while not considering alternative responses to the cues. We hypothesize that some responses are relatively automatic or reflexive, but a given organism can learn to adjust the threshold and timing of response based on the likelihood of a "payoff" as a result of *immediate, delayed, or nonresponse,* and whether the response is a correct one. The animal (or species) without ability to adjust this timing-dependent, payoff-dependent response threshold is less able to adapt to different environments and/or pass its genes on to the next generation. The organism that does not quickly pounce on a potential prey or dodge a potential predator may not get another chance. The relative danger of false-positive responses (e.g., mistaking a neutral cue for a threat and responding defensively) could be easily outweighed by the "downsides" of missing a critical cue in dangerous or resource-scarce environments. In such environments an organism may learn (through early neuroplastic and sculpting processes) to respond with a relatively low threshold for an action response. Yet such "impulsive" hair-trigger responsivity may be less adaptive as the organism moves into other, less time-critical settings over its life course.

NATURE OF ANCESTRAL ENVIRONMENTS

Converging evidence from anthropology and archeology indicates that the human species diverged from forebears by living for a few million years in hunter–gatherer societies. Foraging was essential. Not uncommonly, resources may have been scarce (or at least only intermittently plentiful), and threats abounded. Yet human culture and society have changed dramatically in the last 10,000 years, more rapidly by far than the pace of evolution of the human genome. A lag in remodeling the genome means that our species' brains still retain the propensity to adapt to environmental features as these were before the emergence of recent civilizations. Thus, to understand the behavioral repertoire of modern-day humans, consideration of our ancestral environments is instructive. Relevant to the traits characteristic of persons with ADHD, we suggest that ancestral environments ranged along several continua, including *safe versus not safe, resource-rich versus impoverished,* and *time-optional versus time-critical.* At one end of these three continua (which we term "response-ready"; see Figure 6.1), humans' survival depended on being (1) hypervigilant, including the ability to retrieve and integrate information through all senses at once—somewhat akin to parallel processing; (2) rapid-scanning; (3) quick to pounce (or flee); and (4) motorically

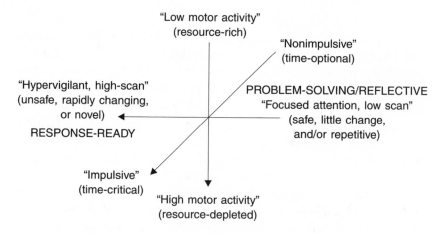

FIGURE 6.1. Dimensions of adaptation related to ADHD-like characteristics.

"hyperactive" (foraging for food, moving toward warmer climes as seasons and ice ages come and go, and so forth). The "response-ready" individual would likely have been advantaged under the brutal or harsh circumstances of the frozen steppe or humid jungle, whereas the excessively contemplative, more phlegmatic individual would have been "environmentally challenged."

Yet not all ancestral environments would have been this harsh, so variability of these traits within the genome would also have been useful for species survival. Within a given hunter–gatherer society, individuals with more of the response-ready characteristics would likely have been successful warriors on a primitive battlefield, whereas those with more contemplative characteristics may have been valued for longer-term planning, strategic operations, or perhaps development of novel solutions to long-standing or even fairly immediate environmental problems. As society has become increasingly industrialized and organized, response-ready characteristics may have become less adaptive, to the extent that current-day environments are more resource-rich, safe, and where a "hair-trigger" time-action response to environmental cues is less critical (even counterproductive). Success in such environments becomes increasingly measured by the ability to demonstrate (1) problem-solving and analytic strategies, (2) restraint of impulsivity, and (3) the controlled deployment of energies. For purposes of our argument, such an individual will be termed "problem-solving."

IS EVERYTHING ADAPTIVE?

Evolutionary adaptational models cannot be all-inclusive, inasmuch as there are likely many pathways though which children elaborate specific behavioral patterns. In some instances ADHD may reflect the effects of perinatal anoxia, maternal cigarette smoke exposure *in utero*, traumatic brain injury, child abuse, or a combination of a host of environmental experiences coupled with susceptibility genes. Yet the importance of an evolutionary model of ADHD rests with its ability to better explain discrepant findings in the research literature; elaborate novel (and testable) hypotheses that shed new light on ADHD phenomena; lead to more effective models of intervention; or clarify the relations between health and disease (Jensen et al., 1997).

CLINICAL IMPLICATIONS

Viewed from an evolutionary, adaptational perspective, our current school environments could hardly be more difficult for the "response-ready" child. Most of them demand attentional focus and motoric passivity, while presenting complex stimuli. They offer many distractions (e.g., large class size), yet funnel information through one modality only, as in passive listening or reading. They limit opportunities for shifting attention and for motor response and demand delay of recognition for efforts. Most school environments favor the "problem-solving" individual, able to maintain intellectual activity with motor quietness, screen out distractions, sustain attention, and delay response until all aspects of a situation have been analyzed. Individual variations along the dimensions of "response-ready" versus "problem-solving" may coincide with environmental variations in a way that produces either a good or bad fit for a particular child. Not surprisingly, many parents and clinicians note that a response-ready child may struggle greatly with a given classroom or teacher, but do much better in another setting, simply through accommodation to the child's abilities (seating placement, smaller classroom size, more hands-on learning opportunities, teacher–pupil rapport). Thus, alterations in the environment may reduce the adaptive strain on a child's nervous system whose set point may be at the other pole from the environment in which the child finds him- or herself. Done systematically and strategically over time, could such interventions modify the response-ready child's biologic substrate and brain–behavior relationships (see, e.g., Baxter et al., 1992)?

In reframing the child with ADHD as response-ready, experience-seeking, or alert and curious, the clinician can counsel the child and family to recognize situations in modern society that might favor such an individual, both in school environments and in future career opportunities such as athlete, air traffic controller, salesperson, soldier, entrepreneur, and the like. The clinician can also "frame" the effects of behavioral treatments as teaching the response-ready child to extend his or her range of skills toward increased task focus, motor and impulse inhibition, self-awareness, and problem solving. In addition, the parent and child can adopt the reasonable goal of assisting the child through school without allowing his or her difficulties in that setting to erode self-esteem and motivation to do well in more adaptive societal niches. The child and parents are encouraged to seek situations and areas of potential success where response-ready traits are more adaptive.

Specialized classroom environments tailored to the response-ready child seem potentially beneficial. Swanson (1992) has described special school classrooms and instructional systems designed to shape children's on-task behaviors and maximize their learning. These systems involve individual and group-based contingencies, the tailoring of assignments to a given child's needs, self-paced computer learning, skill-building, active self-monitoring, and so on. The current premium on "mainstreaming" all children, without regard for a child's personal strengths and weaknesses, seems ill conceived for many children with ADHD, because many children with ADHD experience problematic school and vocational outcomes, partly in response to early adverse school experiences (Richters et al., 1995). Inadequate societal investments in school resources, large classroom sizes, and lack of specific teacher training for response-ready children with ADHD seem likely to perpetuate these difficulties.

In considering treatments for a given child, clinicians should be aware that the child's ADHD "symptoms" may be adaptive in some settings but not others. From this perspective, the complaints of some children and parents that stimulant medications make the child seem too sedated, less social, or "not him- or herself" are understandable. Clinicians should be appropriately cautious when treating one aspect of a child's behavior (e.g., reducing hyperactivity and increasing attention span at school) if the same treatment interferes with the child's functioning in other settings. Such possibilities should not be too quickly discounted, inasmuch as research studies have documented medication effects across a range of environments and situations, such as parent–child interactions (Barkley & Cunningham, 1979) and peer relations (Whalen et al., 1979), and across structured and unstructured school settings (Gadow et al., 1990; Hinshaw, 1991; Hinshaw et al., 1989; Kaplan et al., 1990).

To the extent that we conceptualize ADHD symptoms as traits with adaptive value in specific settings, and that we determine the malleability and environmental triggers of these traits, more specific treatments can be developed that take into account the context dependency of children's symptoms. Furthermore, better awareness of how children's brain systems unfold and consolidate during development may catalyze discovery of novel medications that increase the brain's plasticity to new environmental cues.

An evolutionary perspective on the adaptive nature of children's symptoms should not be confused with a statement against the use of medications or even making a diagnosis. Instead, this perspective draws attention to the need for better assessment of the nature of children's environments, the interactive exchanges between children's behaviors and their environmental fits, and environments' potential adverse sculpting of children's behaviors. Such assessments are necessarily complex, must draw information from multiple sources, and must take the child's environments into account in treatment planning. In many circumstances, medications may be the only available or most effective way to help a given child.

RESEARCH IMPLICATIONS

A major implication of the aforementioned ADHD model suggests that more study of the individual components (attention, motor activity, and impulsivity) as specific traits may be warranted. Breaking the syndrome into its specific behavioral components might more easily allow cross-species comparisons of these traits, with animal and experimental models, including examination of the neurobiological underpinnings of these systems. In addition, more research is needed to explore if, and how, such traits might be beneficial in some settings but nonadaptive in others.

Although "response readiness" may be adaptive in some settings, how should such settings be characterized? As others have noted (Boyce et al., 1998; Jensen & Hoagwood, 1997), a typology of contexts ("environtypes") may facilitate study of the interfaces between organisms and their environments. Conceptualizing environments seems complex, but within an evolutionary framework, this complexity can be reduced by considering the critical functions enabling the organism to survive and thrive. Our three-part characterization of environments as *safe/nonsafe, resource-rich/impoverished,* and *time-optional/time-critical* provides understanding of the adaptive nature of ADHD symptoms in *some* cases. Other environmental descriptors may be needed to understand the potentially adaptive circumstances for symptoms of depression, anxiety syndromes, or conduct disorder.

We need further study of the effects of children's early environments on the development of response-ready traits, as well as the malleability of these characteristics. In this context, what is the impact on children's attentional systems of watching television and playing video games? As compared with many school-related tasks that emphasize logic, sequence, discipline, and detachment, television emphasizes imagery, narrative, immediate gratification, and rapid emotional response (Postman, 1993). When images flash across video screens every few seconds, when children use primarily a passive or reactive form of attention, what attentional skills are being developed? Such questions were raised in recent research by Christakis and colleagues (2004), who reported that hours of young children's television watching were related to parents' later reports of attention problems. Although this research finding was not replicated by another team of investigators using somewhat different methods (Obel et al., 2004), it suggests an important area of further inquiry. Thus, how does passive observation of visual stimuli differ from play activities in which the child directly controls the pace of visual, auditory, and tactile stimuli (e.g., playing with toys in a sandbox or exploring a creek in a neighborhood park)?

We hypothesize that scanning or shifting attentional systems can be "up-regulated" as a function of externally driven stimuli during early development (i.e., set on "high scan"), possibly at the expense of attentional systems for focusing and selecting. A child thus affected is less prepared to cope with attentional tasks such as reading, listening to a story in a quiet circle, or sitting at a desk for long periods of time. "Cohort" effects (increasing prevalence of disorder in later-born generations) have not been demonstrated in the prevalence of ADHD symptomatology, as they have in depressive disorders, both in children and adults, but this possibility as a function of changing societal environments warrants systematic study (Garruto et al., 2004).

If attentional regulatory systems are indeed malleable, we need to determine the periods of greatest plasticity and ascertain which children are most susceptible to up-regulation. Once attentional systems have been up-regulated, does that person or animal continue to select environments that are relatively novel, risky, or otherwise highly stimulating? And does further experience in these settings strengthen or consolidate the biological substrate that led to their selection? Using a combination of functional neuroimaging and greater anatomic specification of the neural systems that subserve these regulatory systems, specific tasks may need to be developed that retrain an attentional, motor, or inhibitory system that is maladapted to environmental demands (e.g., Merzenich et al., 1996; Tallal et al., 1996).

Clearly, it would be incorrect to "romanticize" the child with ADHD as simply mismatched with his or her environment, inasmuch as many (but certainly not all) children with ADHD suffer from impairments across home, school, and neighborhood settings. Furthermore, once we humans began to settle in cities, we certainly had institutions that required children to focus attention, sit passively, and delay response, whether in primitive schools (for the privileged few) or in religious ceremonies. Of note, however, Postman (1993) has indicated that our current schools are a very recent invention, largely in the last 400 years, as a result of the information explosion made possible by the printing press.

Better functional understanding of response-ready traits will enable investigators to study their emergence, persistence, or desistence in longitudinal and environmental contexts. In other words, are there critical tasks in the life of the developing organism for which a given trait is adaptive, but only within a specific time period of the life course of that species? Thus, does impulsivity or excessive motor behavior generally decline over the first two decades of life, because such traits serve an important function early on (e.g., exploration, learning), while the caretaker can provide the necessary protections from radical missteps? For example, in one recent molecular genetic study by an outstanding team of investigators (Ding et al., 2002), one variant of the dopamine-4 receptor gene (DRD4 7R) repeatedly shown to be associated with ADHD (as well as with a variety of impulsive and risk-taking characteristics) was sequenced. Given the complexity of the mutational events that would have been required to allow this gene variant to emerge, this team concluded that it could only have arisen in its current frequency in the human species through "positive selection," that is, through some adaptive aspects associated with this allele that it endowed on humans.

A better understanding of the specific traits associated with ADHD may require additional anthropological studies and cross-cultural comparisons in order to determine when such characteristics might be useful. Although ADHD has been described in most Western societies, actual differences in prevalence are unknown, particularly in non-Western societies (Bird et al., 2002). We urge cross-cultural studies of the effects of cultural and environmental factors as they shape the expression of various ADHD-like traits.

Our hypothetical model of why some children might be at risk for developing ADHD, or at least for increased expression of inattentive, hyperactive, or impulsive traits, suggests that more studies of the boundaries between illness and health are needed, as well as what constitutes a "disorder." Indeed, recent findings from the largest genetic twin study of ADHD conducted to date suggest that ADHD is best characterized as a trait distributed normally throughout the population (Levy et al., 1997; Rasmussen et al., 2002). But at which point should a mismatch between persons and environments be designated as a medical psychiatric disorder, particularly when neuroscience findings are increasingly blurring the boundaries between normal and abnormal? As we expand our scientific knowledge, pressure for "medicalizing" many manifestations of human distress may increase and may be seen as beneficent, particularly if society is willing to pay only for "medical" illnesses and not for what are perceived as "problems in living" (Sadler et al., 1994).

In a series of articles Wakefield and colleagues (1992a, 1992b, 2002) have elaborated the construct of "harmful dysfunction," which focuses on the identification of a pathological process or function per se, as well as the determination that this pathophysiological process within the individual results in some impairment or harm for that individual within a given society. Both components (harm *and* dysfunction) must be present to identify a mental disorder. This promising approach may, nevertheless, present problems to the extent that a "dysfunction" of a natural process cannot be understood outside the context in which the function evolved. Some presumed biological dysfunctions are best conceptualized as the displacement of the organism from its original ecological niche.

We suggest that evolutionary biology provides a useful framework for understanding ADHD, and possibly a range of psychiatric phenomena, just as it does for almost all areas of medicine. Our proposed hypotheses are testable through cross-cultural and cross-species comparisons, experimental animal models, and various research strategies appropriate and generally accepted among evolutionary scientists. Although these ideas may seem speculative or simply wrong by some (Brody, 2001), Popper has suggested that new ideas must be nursed, particularly when one paradigm becomes too dominant, too much like a monopoly, or an entrenched ideology—a "fashion of science" (Popper, 1994). In the case of ADHD, where the current ideology is supported by the scientific infrastructure and by economic incentives (treatment programs, school systems, and the pharmaceutical industry), attempts toward progress may not always be welcome. However, as new theory, these ideas can lead to different hypotheses and novel study approaches (Andrews et al., 2002), as compared with the currently dominant theories. Understanding ADHD symptoms within the context of their adaptive functions is a promising alternative strategy for discovering and understanding gene–environment and brain–behavior interactions and offers the eventual possibility to develop more effective preventive and treatment interventions.

ACKNOWLEDGMENT

This chapter was adapted from Jensen et al. (1997). Copyright 1997 by Lippincott Williams & Wilkins. Adapted by permission.

REFERENCES

Andrews PW, Gangestad SW, Matthews D (2002). Adaptationism—How to carry out an exaptationist program. *Behav Brain Sci*, 25:489–504.
Barkley RA & Cunningham CE (1979) The effects of methylphenidate on the mother–child interactions of hyperactive children. *Arch Gen Psychiatry*, 36:201–208.

Baxter LR, Schwartz JM, Bergman KS, Szuba MP, Guze BH, Massiotta JC, Alazraki A, Selin CE, Ferng HK, Munford P, & Phelps ME (1992) Caudate glucose metabolic rate changes with both drug and behavior therapy for obsessive–compulsive disorder. *Arch Gen Psychiatry,* 49:681–689.

Bird HR (2002) The diagnostic classification, epidemiology, and cross-cultural validity of ADHD. In PS Jensen & JR Cooper (Eds.), *Attention-deficit hyperactivity disorder: State of science—best practices* (pp. 2.1–2.16). Kingston, NJ: Civic Research Institute.

Bowlby J (1973) *Attachment and loss: Vol. 2. Separation.* New York: Basic Books.

Boyce WT, Frank E, Jensen PS, Kessler RC, Nelson CA, & Steinberg L (1998) The role of context in developmental psychopathology: A theoretical perspective from the MacArthur Network on Psychopathology and Development. *Dev Psychopathology,* 10:143–164.

Brody JF (2001) Evolutionary recasting: ADHD, mania and its variants (2001). *J Affective Disord,* 65(2):197–215.

Christakis DA, Zimmerman FJ, DiGiuseppe DL, & McCarty CA (2004) Early television exposure and subsequent attentional problems in children. *Pediatrics,* 113:708 –713.

Ding YC, Chi HC, Grady DL, Morishima A, Kidd JR, Kidd KK, Flodman P, Spence MA, Schuck S, Swanson JM, Zhang YP, & Moyzis RK (2002) Evidence of positive selection acting at the human dopamine receptor D4 gene locus. *Proc Nat Acad Sci U.S.A.,* 99:309–314.

Gadow KD, Nolan EE, Sverd J, Sprafkin J, & Paolicelli L (1990) Methylphenidate in aggressive–hyperactive boys: I. Effects on peer aggression in public school settings. *J Am Acad Child Adolesc Psychiatry,* 29:710–718.

Garruto RM, Little MA, & Weitz CA (2004) Environmental stress and adaptational responses: Consequences for human health outcomes. *Coll Antropol,* 28:509–540.

Hinshaw SP (1991) Stimulant medication and the treatment of aggression in children with attentional deficits. *J Clin Child Psychol,* 15:301–312.

Hinshaw SP, Buhrmester D, & Heller T (1989) Anger control in response to verbal provocation: Effects of stimulant medication for boys with ADHD. *J Abnorm Child Psychol,* 17:393–407.

Jensen PS & Hoagwood K (1997) The book of names: DSM-IV in context. *Dev Psychopathology,* 9:231–249.

Jensen PS, Mrazek D, Knapp PK, Steinberg L, Pfeffer C, Schowalter J, & Shapiro T (1997) Evolution and revolution included psychiatry: ADHD as a disorder of adaptation. *J Am Acad Child Adolesc Psychiatry,* 36(12):1672–1679.

Kaplan SL, Busner J, Kupooetz S, Wassermann E, & Segal B (1990) Effects of methylphenidate on adolescents with aggressive conduct disorder and

ADDH: A preliminary report. *J Am Acad Child Adolesc Psychiatry*, 29:719–723.

Levy F, Hay DA, McStephen M, Wood C, & Waldman I (1997) Attention-deficit hyperactivity disorder: A category or a continuum? Genetic analysis of a large-scale twin study. *J Am Acad Child Adolesc Psychiatry*, 36:737–744.

Lima SL & Dill LM (1990) Behavioral decisions made under the risk of predation: A review and prospectus. *Can J Zool,* 68: 619–640.

Merzenich MM, Jenkins WM, Johnston P, Schreiner C, Miller SL, & Tallal P (1996) Temporal processing deficits of language-learning impaired children ameliorated by training. *Science*, 271:77–81.

Obel C, Henriksen TB, Dalsgaard S, Linnet KM, Skajaa E, Thomsen PH, & Olsen J (2004) Does children's watching of television cause attention problems? Retesting the hypothesis in a Danish cohort. *Pediatrics*, 114(5):1372–1373.

Popper KR (1994) *The myth of the framework: In defense of science and rationality.* New York: Routledge.

Postman N (1993) *Technopoly: The surrender of culture to technology.* New York: Vintage Books.

Rasmussen ER, Neuman RJ, Heath AC, Levy F, Hay DA, & Todd RD (2002) Replication of the latent class structure of attention-deficit/hyperactivity disorder (ADHD) subtypes in a sample of Australian twins. *J Child Psychol Psychiatry*, 43:1018–1028.

Richters J, Arnold LEA, Jensen PS, Abikoff H, Conners CK, Greenhill L, Hechtman L, Hinshaw S, Pelham W, & Swanson J (1995) NIMH collaborative multisite, multimodal treatment study of children with ADHD: I. Background and rationale. *J Am Acad Child Adolesc Psychiatry*, 34:987–1000.

Sadler JZ, Wiggins OP, & Schwartz MA (1994) Introduction. In JZ Sadler, OP Wiggins, & MA Schwartz (Eds.), *Philosophical perspectives on psychiatric diagnostic classification*, (pp. 1–13). Baltimore: Johns Hopkins University Press.

Shibagaki M & Yamanaka T (1990) Attention of preschool children: Electrodermal activity during auditory stimulation. *Percept Motor Skills*, 70:207–215.

Swanson JM (1992) *School-based assessments and interventions for ADD students.* Irvine, CA: K.C. Publishing.

Tallal P, Miller SL, Bedi G, Byma G, Wang X, Nagarajan SS, Schreiner C, Jenkins WM, & Merzenich MM (1996) Language comprehension in language learning impaired children improved with acoustically modified speech. *Science*, 271:81–84.

Wakefield JC (1992a) Disorder as harmful dysfunction: A conceptual critique of DSM-III-R's definition of mental disorder. *Psychol Rev*, 99:232–247.

Wakefield JC (1992b) The concept of mental disorder: On the boundary between biological facts and social values. *Am Psychol*, 47:373–388.

Wakefield JC, Pottick KJ, & Kirk SA (2002) Should the DSM-IV diagnostic criteria for conduct disorder consider social context? *Am J Psychiatry* 159:380–386.

Werner EE & Anholt B (1993) Ecological consequences of the tradeoff between growth and mortality rates mediated by foraging activity. *Am Naturalist*, 142:242–272.

Whalen CK, Henker B, Collins BE, McAuliffe S, & Vaux A (1979) Peer interaction in a structured communication task: Comparisons of normal and hyperactive boys and of methylphenidate (Ritalin) and placebo effects. *Child Dev*, 50:388–401.

CHAPTER 7

Conduct Disorder
and Evolutionary Biology

MARKUS KRUESI *and* JOHN SCHOWALTER

This chapter considers the relationships of evolutionary biology to the diagnosis conduct disorder (CD) and its neurobiology. One form of CD is particularly likely to relate to an evolutionary perspective: the subtype that "breeds true" and grows into antisocial personality disorder (ASP). Although childhood conduct disturbance is common, less than half of such instances persist into adulthood (Rutter, 1989). In contrast, ASP is almost always preceded by CD in childhood (Robins, 1966, 1978). This chapter focuses on CD and its continuity with ASP.

Aggression and criminality/delinquency are related but not entirely the same concepts. However, many studies use these terms interchangeably with conduct disorder/antisocial personality with confusing results and implications. Aggression has considerable overlap with conduct disorder, but there are individuals with conduct disorder who do not display aggression. *Delinquency* is a legal term. Juvenile delinquents may present with no diagnosis at all or with many different diagnoses (Quay, 1979). Prevalence data for adult ASP and for juvenile delinquency provide useful referents in attempting to interpolate from studies using those noninterchangeable diagnoses. Antisocial personality disorder in adults had a lifetime prevalence of 0.8% for females and 4.5% for males in the Epidemiologic Catchment Area study (Robins et al., 1991). In contrast, juvenile delinquency has far higher prevalence rates, as 65% of male adolescents self-report lawbreaking and 25% have experienced police contact or arrest (Farrington et al., 1986).

This most recent version of criteria for CD tightened the operational definition of the disorder and appears to be more consistent with ASP. Sociopathy is often used as a synonym for ASP. The previous DSM-III-R symptom "often lies" was dropped and replaced by a more specific operational definition: "often lies or breaks promises to obtain goods or favors from others (i.e., 'cons' others)." This focus on intent to "con" others appears consistent with ASP. Test–retest agreement and internal consistency for the CD diagnosis have improved with the DSM-IV version (Lahey et al., 1994). DSM-IV recognizes that childhood onset, defined as the presence of one or more CD symptoms prior to age 10, is at increased risk of proceeding to ASP.

As Pine and Shapiro point out in their chapter on anxiety disorders (Chapter 4), there is relatively little genetic variability in traits carrying a strong selective advantage, for if a trait is highly adaptive, the forces of natural selection create population homogeneity. So how is it that antisocial personality persists in the human population? A look at the evolutionary roots of CD provides a useful starting point.

All evolutionary theories must be speculative. Rule breaking is no exception, particularly since we know little about what rules were extant before Hammurabi's code in Babylon of the 18th century B.C. and the Ten Commandments, handed down through Moses in the 13th century B.C. It does not, however, seem too much of a reach to assume that murder has made every list of rules, no matter when or where it was drawn up. Cain's murder of Abel is cited in Genesis as an example of original sin. As that murder forewarned, it is very possible that male violence has topped disease and famine as the overall greatest scourge of civilization. Now that there are weapons of mass destruction, violence is the most likely way that civilization will be ended. Along with the Ten Commandments, Moses, also in the book of Exodus, codifies violence for violence: "And if any mischief follow, then thou shalt give life for life, eye for eye, tooth for tooth, hand for hand, foot for foot, burning for burning, wound for wound, stripe for stripe" (Exodus 21:23–25). Violence is clearly the easiest antisocial conduct to track over the millennia.

Darwin suggested, "Multiply, vary, let the strongest live and the weakest die" (1859). He believed the three basic human emotions to be anger, rage, and fear—what we now think of as keystones for fight or flight. As we do today, Darwin (1872) thought that the seats of emotions in the brain are primitive and date from early evolution. Darwin (1871) speculated that early humans lived in small groups in which the strongest male drove off all male rivals for his wives and daughters. Freud (1953b) hypothesized as a stereotype that at some time rusticated young males banded together, returned, and killed the primal male. This action, among other things, freshened the gene pool. All evidence suggests that personal violence was more crucial in prehistoric time than now. Before "equalizer" distance weapons such as arrows and guns, personal strength and cunning were paramount in spreading a male's genes in what was almost always a polygynous society. This breeding wrought a genetic system within which the fitness of males was more favored than the fitness of females. Qualities helpful in combat were passed on selectively.

In earliest times, a male's prowess as a hunter was of great significance. Interestingly, as farming gained importance, so did the ownership and protection of land. This brought forth more human-to-human violence. A warrior class arose to defend people's own accumulations and to plunder other groups' lands and accumulations. Through the subsequent ages in most cultures, warrior values became the accepted values of maleness. Violence is typically resorted to when territories are limited, one's offspring are threatened, food is scarce, and in the context of competitive mating (Archer, 1988). Until the 19th century, armies were usually not paid wages; their pay was agreed to be rape and pillage. This practice further spread particular genetic traits.

The most common symptom associated with antisocial personality disorder, as reported by all three sites of the Epidemiologic Catchment Area Project, was fighting (Robins, 1985). From earlier studies we already know that aggression among individuals over time has a stability that rivals that of intellectual ability, while also over time being a robust predictor of antisocial behavior (Huesmann et al., 1984; Olweus, 1972). Aggression, however, need not always be destructive and rule breaking. When used, for example, effectively within societal or athletic rules, it is likely to enhance an individual's self-esteem and status. It seems clear in the 21st century that aggressive potential is in all of us, some more than others, particularly in males. The quality of a person's aggression is what is important. When the quality of aggression leads to conduct and antisocial disorders, social status is likely to fall. Low status, we know, at least in primates, is likely to lower serotonin (Raleigh & McGuire, 1991) and in humans to lower testosterone (Gladue et al., 1989). Such biological changes are likely to further a downward slide in self-esteem and status. Antisocial personality disorder also tends to lead to earlier deaths, mainly through drug use, suicide, and homicide (Rutter et al., 1998). However, again particularly for males, the use of assertiveness, if not aggression, to successfully enhance social status may lead to higher levels of testosterone, possibly higher levels of serotonin (Raleigh & McGuire, 1991), and, for sure, longer life (Marmot & Shipley, 1996).

Fighting is not the only means of gaining power or of passing on one's genes. Historically, the formation of larger and larger human groups probably tempered the unique importance of male violence. Rules were more likely to be drawn and enforced. "Behavior, not thought or emotion, is what natural selection passes judgement on" (Wright, 1995). The two, not mutually exclusive, male behaviors that are most likely to garner high status and resources in a society are those that elicit fear of one's ability and willingness to cause harm and those that elicit desirableness of one's ability and willingness to protect others. If successful, the first leader takes what he wants and the second is given what he wants. With the march of civilization, reproductive success increasingly required social, as well as combative, prowess. Though it is true that species and cultures that function well without competition are extremely rare, leaders' reputations are made at times of crisis, and sometimes competitions are not worth the resources that will be lost through the battle. Leadership and judgment became progressively desirable as societies became large and complex. No one can survive unless he or she, alone or with help, is able to escape danger. Genes that promote flexibility of behavior ultimately lead to more successful adaptation than genes that support inflexible behaviors, such as the drive to fight even when faced with certain disastrous failure. This is true for both leaders and other individuals. Fighters are forced to be winners or losers, and losers often lose both life and the chance for progeny. Because the overall human gene pool, regardless of country or society, is essentially identical to what it was at the beginning of written history, the rules and environmental teachings of a culture or subculture greatly influence how the emotions of anger, fear, and rage are expressed. Well-functioning societies and persons have goals. Aggression and violence may be strategies, but they in themselves are not goals. Rules, for the most part, are protection from unfair aggression and violence. Angry people want to take, not cooperate. Conduct disorder and antisocial personality disorder are not, however, caused only by problems within the individual but, more accurately, by problems between the individual and society. The more unfair laws a society has, the more lawbreakers it will produce, particularly if the society does not show consistency and vigor in raising children to follow rules and/or does not mete out punishment consistently and fairly. "Predisposition is not predestination" (Hamer & Copeland, 1999), but although genes do not cause a teenager to commit crimes, they may make a youngster supersensitive to a wrong environment and may influence the likelihood that he or she will be in the wrong place at the wrong time (Cadoret et al., 1995; Rutter et al., 1999). Scarr and McCartney (1983) pointed out the importance of the interaction between gene and environment. In fact, already in 1905, Freud (1953a) taught that "the constitutional factor must await experience before it can make itself felt; the accidental factor must have a constitutional basis in order to come into operation."

Leckman and Mayes (1998) have made clear that principles from evolutionary biology can be one useful source for understanding developmental psychopathology. They also warn that actually proving specific evolutionary theories may be impossible. This is certainly true. Nonetheless, the thread of males' violent rule breaking—from the time of humankind's earliest rule givers, through the ebbs and flows of various civilizations, to the 1899 creation of a juvenile court in Chicago that led to the formation of child psychiatry as a medical discipline, to the establishment of DSM criteria for conduct disorder and antisocial personality disorder, to the current state in which violence is a major behavior leading to childrens' and adolescents' admissions to psychiatric hospitals—is a very strong thread indeed.

Aggression forms an important set of criteria for the diagnosis of CD/ASP. But not all aggression is part of conduct disorder, and aggression may not be the only aspect of conduct disorder with an evolutionary role. Two major types of aggression, predatory and affective, have long been recognized to have neurobiological contrasts

(Kruesi et al., 2003). Neither type is exclusive to CD/ASP. For example, both strong-arm robbery and hunting deer as a food source qualify as predatory aggression. But in many locales only the first would be viewed as antisocial behavior. The inappropriate nature and modulation of aggression are often the salient features. For example, cruelty can make an aggressive action qualify for CD/ASP. As strong a thread as violence is, evolutionary biology assigns a premium to the actual passage of genes. Although selective pressure and/or violence may limit the availability of certain genes, the transmission of genes has until quite recently required reproductive behavior.

An early attempt to address the evolutionary biological fit of ASP was a seminal paper by MacMillan and Kofoed (1984). MacMillan and Kofoed proposed that ASP, in sociobiological terms, represented an alternate reproductive strategy—a minimal investment reproductive strategy. Those authors pointed to a continuum of reproductive strategies that range from a maximal investment, characterized by protracted care of the young and minimal numbers of offspring, to a minimal investment strategy characterized by lack of care for the young and greater numbers of offspring. Larger numbers of offspring, more promiscuous matings (Robins, 1966), more abuse/neglect/abandonment of partners and offspring (Robins, 1966), and a "cheating" reproductive strategy whereby males misrepresent their position in the dominance heirarchy to mate were cited by MacMillan and Kofoed as evidence of that alternate strategy. In contrast, nonantisocial individuals were said to be more likely to have a greater investment/fewer offspring strategy. The Robins (1966) data, published in *Deviant Children Grown Up,* provided evidence that even as compared with individuals with other psychiatric disorders, those with ASP were significantly more likely to have a greater number of sexual partners and to have abandoned/abused/neglected their offspring and mates.

Rolls (1999), in discussing sexual behavior, reward, and brain function, wrote, "In the long term, once sociobiologic hypotheses have have been presented, they must be tested." The sections that follow seek to examine the evidence for the hypothesis that antisocial personality, and hence the CD that preceeds it, constitute an alternate reproductive adaptation.

Subsequent to Robins's (1966) work, later investigations and reviews amplified and added to Robins's landmarks and offered additional documentation that the reproductive adaptation of antisocial individuals differs from that of others. The observation that "prostitution is frequent among female sociopaths, and homosexual prostitution is common among male sociopaths" (Goodwin & Guze, 1979) supports the notion of greater numbers of partners relative to the general population.

Having a greater number of sexual partners appears to be a characteristic of the reproductive adaptation of antisocial individuals. A fair amount of consistency is seen even when the presence of other comorbid conditions that may be associated with different sexual behavior are controlled for. In a study of 154 psychiatric patients, antisocial personality was associated with increased numbers of sexual partners (Spalt, 1975). More recently, HIV infection and/or the risk of HIV infection prompted a number of researchers to explore relationships between ASP in substance abusers and HIV risk behaviors (Tourian et al., 1997). Sexual risk behaviors are associated with greater seroconversion rates. Consequent to such studies we have more data about the sexual behavior of antisocial persons, as well as evidence that the difference in sexual behavior exists when the potential confound between substance abuse and ASP is controlled for. Again, the picture of a significantly greater number of sexual partners is generally seen. A study of 55 methadone patients found that those with ASP were significantly more likely to be promiscuous—defined as having 10 or more sexual partners in the past year (Gill et al., 1992). A separate study of 351 cocaine abusers also found that those with ASP are more promiscuous, using the same definition in the Gill and colleagues study (Compton et al., 1995). Tourian and colleagues (1997) did not find those with ASP to be more likely to have multiple sex partners in their study of 289 opiate-dependent methadone patients. However, the Tourian study used a definition of more than 1 partner in the past 6 months to operationalize the category "multiple sex partners." Therefore, it may be that this less stringent definition of larger versus smaller number of sexual partners obscured a finding. A recent birth cohort study of 930 New Zealand residents found antisocial persons to have an odds ratio of 2.4 for intercourse with 3 or more partners in the last year with whom condoms are not used regularly (Ramrakha et al., 2000). In that study, the risky nature of these sexual encounters is evident in the increased risk ratio for sexually transmitted disease.

Another consistent finding is assortative mating among sociopathic individuals; they tend to mate with other sociopathic individuals (Cloninger & Guze, 1970; Guze et al., 1970; Krueger et al., 1998). A study of 360 couples from Dunedin, New Zealand, found substantial assortative mating in self-reports of antisocial behavior per se and in self-reports of couple members' tendencies to associate with antisocial peers: 0.54 on average (Krueger et al., 1998). Perceptions about the likelihood of social sanctions for antisocial behavior (e.g., being caught by the authorities or losing the respect of one's family) showed moderately associative mating (0.32 on average). However, assortative mating for personality traits related to antisocial behavior was low (0.15 on average). These findings suggest that, whereas assortative mating for many individual difference variables (such as personality traits) is low, assortative mating for actual antisocial behaviors is substantial. Although assortative mating runs high among antisocial individuals, a critical question is whether the nonassortative matings of individuals with CD/ASP is more varied (dissimilar in a genetic sense) than the nonassortative matings of nonantisocial individuals. If the nonassortative matings of antisocial individuals are more genetically varied than those of nonantisocial individuals, then it argues for an evolutionary role for CD/ASP in "stirring" or mixing the gene pool.

Studies of the sexual behavior of juveniles are less frequent; nonetheless, such studies also suggest that the reproductive adaptation of indviduals with CD/ASP, as manifested by their sexual behavior and childrearing practices, differs from that of others. Individuals with ASP were recognized to begin heterosexual exeriences earlier than others and much more likely to be indiscriminate in their sexual behavior (Goodwin and Guze, 1979). Early sexual initiation has long been associated with "problem behaviors" in adolescence (Jessor & Jessor, 1977; Stewart et al., 1980). More recently, because of the increasingly earlier onset of penetrative sexual activities, investigators have begun examining the sexual behavior of middle childhood. A study of 126 boys ages 5–11 years at increased risk for the development of CD-related behavior revaluated 112 of them 15 months later (Meyer-Bahlburg et al., 1999). At both time points, the boys scored higher on the Sex Problems scale as well as on the nonsexual Child Behavior Check List (CBCL) scales than Achenbach's nonclinical norm sample. Within the at-risk sample, the Sex Problems scale was significantly related to externalizing problem behaviors, but also to the other CBCL scales of behavioral/emotional problems. Data analyzed from 5,877 respondents ages 15–54 years in the National

Comorbidity Survey, a nationally representative household survey, indicated that early-onset psychiatric disorders were associated with subsequent teenage parenthood among both females and males, with significant odds ratios of 2.0–12.0 and population attributable risk proportions of 6.2–33.7% (Kessler et al., 1997). Because of this risk, due to the general category of early-onset psychiatric disorder, it is important that studies address psychiatric comorbidity in order to parse out relationships to CD.

Recent studies have shed light on the association between CD and sexual/reproductive behavior by controlling for confounds. Girls with CD, girls with depression, girls with anxiety, and healthy girls ($n = 459$) who had been evaluated at age 15 years were followed up at age 21, when reproductive health was assessed (Bardone et al., 1998). After control for potentially confounding variables including prior health, adolescent CD predicted more medical problems, poorer self-reported overall health, lower body mass index, alcohol and/or marijuana dependence, tobacco dependence, daily smoking, more lifetime sexual partners, sexually transmitted disease, and early pregnancy. In a separate study, 83 girls, ages 8–13 years, at study entry with childhood-onset psychiatric disorders were repeatedly evaluated during an interval of up to 12 years (Kovacs et al., 1994). In the final model, childhood- or adolescent-onset conduct disorders (but not depressive disorders) were significantly associated with teenage pregnancy. Among the girls with conduct disorders, 54.8% became pregnant teenagers versus 12% of the rest. In addition to earlier sexual initiation, pregnancy, and greater numbers of partners, there are indications that other aspects of sexuality differ as well. A recent birth cohort study of 930 New Zealand residents found that individuals with ASP have a risk ratio of 2.8 for early-onset intercourse (prior to age 16), whereas those with depressive disorders have a risk ratio of 1.3 (Ramrakha et al., 2000). This is consistent with the idea that it is CD that is driving the early age of sexual initiation rather than other psychiatric disorders.

Sexual victimization, as victim or as perpetrator, is associated with CD in both clinical and community samples. A study of 1,025 females and 1,087 males in grades 7–12 in Alberta (Canada) high schools found associations between experiencing a high number of sexual assaults and clinical profiles on measures of conduct disorder for both males and females (Bagley et al., 1995). Conduct disorder was present in 94% of a clinical sample of 17 adolescents who sexually molested children (Galli et al., 1999). In a study of 499 mentally ill children and adolescents that grouped subjects in four mutually exclusive categories—no inappropriate sexual behavior ($n = 296$), hypersexual ($n = 82$), exposing ($n = 39$), and victimizing ($n = 82$)—an antisocial family history was associated with increased rates of sexually inappropriate behaviors (Adams et al., 1995). One criterion symptom for conduct disorder is "has forced someone into sexual activity" (DSM-IV), therefore the "victimizing" group might be expected to be associated with antisocial family histories. However, hypersexuality and exposing behaviors were also associated with antisocial family histories, suggesting that antisocial family history is associated with a broad range of sexual behaviors that differ in qualitative and quantitative ways from those of other youth.

Another facet of reproductive adaptation, parenting or care of the young, also differs between antisocial and other families—those with ASP tend to have less parental monitoring, greater family conflict, and lower family involvement (Ary et al., 1999; Patterson et al., 1989). The predictive association between parenting and adolescent adjustment has been assumed to be environmental. However, one recent examination of genetic and environmental contributions suggests a need for greater consideration of genetic contributions. A study of 395 families with adolescent siblings who participated in the Nonshared Environment in Adolescent Development (Reiss et al., 1994) project at two times of assessment, 3 years apart. There were five sibling types in two types of families: 63 identical twins, 75 fraternal twins, and 58 full siblings in nondivorced families, and 95 full, 60 half, and 44 genetically unrelated siblings in stepfamilies. Results indicate that the cross-lagged associations between parental conflict negativity and adolescent antisocial behavior can be explained primarily by genetic factors (Neiderhiser et al., 1999).

Reproductive adaptation is a behaviorally expressed function associated with neuroanatomic differences, as has been demonstrated among progressively more closely related specimens. Comparison of the orders Insectivora (moles, shrews, which feed on insects) and Edentata (armadillos, tree sloths, anteaters) revealed that larger brain size was associated with a reproductive adaptation marked by increased lifespan, smaller litter size, and protracted parental care of the young (Eisenberg, 1981). In congeneric species of voles with contrasting reproductive strategies (polygamous versus monogamous), parental and affiliative behaviors differ in terms of relative hippocampal volume (Jacobs et al., 1990) and cell density of the anteroventral-periventricular nucleus (Shapiro et al., 1991). Within the species plainfish midshipman (*Porichthys notatus*), a sound-producing teleost fish, there exist two alternate mating strategies among males. Type I males vocalize to attract females to the nests that the males have built and then guard the eggs until the embryos hatch and swim free. Type II males neither build nests nor vocally attract females but "sneak" spawn—fertilizing the eggs in the nest of another male. A seminal study of the two alternate types of males found that intrasexual dimorphism of vocal motor phenotypes, such as the dimensions of vocal neurons, accompanies the divergence of reproductive traits (Bass, 1992). Subsequent work by the same group found that sexual differentiation of the vocal motor system in the midshipman begins early in development, well before any evidence of sexual maturation (Knapp et al., 1999). Thus, one might expect neuroanatomic differences between individuals with ASP and other humans. How gross or subtle might the differences be?

Brain volume differences are said to follow the principle of "proper mass," wherein closely related species that emphasize one function over another have relatively more brain tissue devoted to the more dominant function (Jerison, 1973, 1988). For example, Kruska (1988) pointed out that in the process of domestication of the European boar into the domestic pig, receptor cells in the eye's retina (Wigger, 1939), as well as in the olfactory epithelium (Guntherschulze, 1979), are reduced in number to a degree comparable to the decrease in size of brain structures (Kruska, 1980). Keen senses needed for hunting are not necessary in the domesticated pig. In an analogous manner, there is a volumetric increase in the vocal motor neuron volume in Type I male teleost fish with sexual maturity, which is not seen in Type II males (Bass et al., 1996). The Type I males generate long-duration advertisement calls to attract females to a nest, whereas the Type II males sneak-spawn and, like females, do not produce mate calls but generate short-duration agonistic calls. Thus, following the principle of proper mass, it is logical that Type II males, because they do not need to vocalize to mate, would not have as large a vocal motor neuron volume as the other reproductive morph.

Neuroanatomic differences between males of the same species with differing reproductive adaptations led Kruesi and colleagues (1993, 2004) to hypothesize that neuroanatomic differences would be present in comparing individuals at high risk for ASP with those who are not at risk for the disorder. Regional brain volumes were assessed from magnetic resonance imaging (MRI) scans in 10 patients with early-onset CD (nine males and one female) at high risk for ASP and compared with 10 age-, sex-, and handedness-matched control children. Because it utilized relatively primitive MRI volumetric techniques, the investigation was limited to whole and regional brain volumes. This generation of MRI volumetric analysis represented a search for nonsubtle differences and was likened to "dissecting the brain with a snow shovel." Two regions were targeted for examination: the prefrontal and temporal regions. Right temporal lobe volumes were significantly smaller in individuals with CD at high risk for ASP, as compared with controls, even when trends for smaller total brain volumes were controlled for. Prefrontal volumes were smaller in the group at high risk for ASP, but not significantly so. Raine and colleagues, in a study with more recent measurement technology and a larger number of participants, found significantly smaller frontal gray matter volumes in 21 males with ASP, as compared with control groups: 34 healthy volunteers, 26 substance abusers, and 21 psychiatric controls (Raine et al., 2000). Unfortunately, Raine and colleagues did not address temporal lobe volumes. However, the Raine and colleagues (2000) study examined autonomic activity during a stressful task and decreased autonomic activity in the antisocial group. Because the prefrontal cortex is part of a neural circuit that plays a role in stress reactivity (Frysztak & Neafsey, 1994) and fear conditioning (Hugdahl, 1998), the poor conditioning and less autonomic reactivity during aversive stimuli are hypothesized mechanisms that fit the anatomic deficit and may predispose an individual to ASP (Raine et al., 2000).

In summary, there is a growing and substantial consistency of evidence to support the idea that ASP represents an alternate reproductive adaptation among humans. There appears consistent support for those with ASP differing in their number of sexual partners and for their comparative lack of investment in their young.

However, there are other aspects of reproductive behavior that would be consistent with the hypothesis that ASP is a different reproductive adaptation that have not been assessed. MacMillan and Kofoed (1984) pointed out that individuals with ASP are also more apt than others to fail to mate. This they attributed to the low position of males with ASP in the dominance heirarchy and their resultant unattractiveness to females. Thus, individuals with ASP need to misrepresent their position in the dominance heirarchy in order to mate. MacMillan and Kofoed referred to this as a "cheating" reproductive strategy.

There are incentives for females to choose both males who will invest in their offspring and males who appear attractive and dominant (even if they do not invest in the offspring). The former contribute to evolutionary fitness, or the transmission of genes to succeeding generations, by helping care for and support the young who have a prolonged period of time to mature. But a wife (or her genes) also benefits by obtaining genes as fit as possible, sometimes by cheating on her husband (Rolls, 1999). Studies of human paternity show that the father is misidentified in about 14% of cases (Baker & Bellis, 1995; Ridley, 1993). A key question is whether ASP is overrepresented in that 14% of those of deceptive paternity.

In addition, one might hypothesize that males successfully using a "cheating" reproductive strategy might have certain sexual characteristics in addition to a general ability to deceive. For this to be an efficient strategy, males with ASP who mate nonassortatively would benefit from being efficient at mating. Because deception becomes progressively harder to maintain over time, it would be of benefit to have an increased conception rate among matings by cheaters (and those with ASP). Based on questionnaire data, Baker and Bellis (1995) found that in unfaithful women having sex with their husbands, only 45% of the copulations were of the high-retention type, but 70% of the copulations with the lover were of the orgasmic high-retention type more likely to result in conception. In contrast, 55% of the copulations of faithful women were of the most fertile high-retention type. One interpretation is that this phenomenon appears to represent the ability of a woman, to some extent, to influence who the father of her children will be, not only by having sex with her lover but also by influencing whether she conceives by that lover (Rolls, 1999). A corollary, for which we were unable to find any data in the literature, is that males with ASP would be predicted to have greater efficacy in getting females to orgasm, which would result in "upsuck" and greater retention of sperm. Given the need for deception, with dissimilar partners mating frequency would be apt to be less often than for those in stable relationships. Therefore, a more reliable production of orgasm would be advantageous.

Another aspect of reproductive adaptation and efficiency of mating concerns twinning, especially dizygotic twin births. If multiple egg production is part of a greater numbers, lesser investment strategy, then certain facts may be ordered (Rushton, 1987). Twin births are more efficient for passing on genes because more are passed on per pregnancy. This would be expected to be particularly important for females with ASP. Given their increased risk of sexually transmitted disease and attendant loss of fertility, increased twin rates would be desirable for females with ASP. Some view increased dizygotic twinning as evidence of a decreased investment reproductive strategy (Rushton, 1987), which would add consistency to the MacMillan and Kofoed (1984) assertion. Many comparisons between mothers of singletons and mothers of dizygotic (DZ) twins by Rushton (1987) would appear to parallel comparisons between antisocial females and their non-ASP counterparts. As compared with mothers of singletons, for example, mothers of DZ twins have a lower age of menarche, a shorter menstrual cycle, a greater number of marriages, a higher rate of coitus, more illegitimate children, a closer spacing of births, greater fecundity, more wasted pregnancies, larger families, earlier menopause, and earlier mortality. Furthermore, all twins have a shorter gestation period, a lower birth weight, and a greater incidence of infant mortality, with DZ twins having a greater frequency of health disorders, a higher mortality rate, and a lower rate of enrollment in volunteer registries. Multiple birthing also occurs more frequently in families of lower than of higher social status, and in those of African descent more than in those of European, or, especially, those of Asian descent. This ethnic difference is *not* consistent with the epidemiology of ASP, because rates of ASP were similar in European Americans and African Americans despite the overrepresentation of African Americans among prison populations (Robins et al., 1991). Nonetheless, the prediction is that one would find increased twinning among females with ASP. A search of the literature turned up no data to answer the question of whether females with ASP have increased rates of twinning.

Generally, the evidence thus far supports the hypothesis that ASP is a different reproductive adaptation. But an unanswered question is why should two different reproductive adaptations coexist in a given species. One possibility is the additional adaptive capacity this offers for the species. Certain conditions may favor individuals with ASP, and under certain circumstances there may be a survival benefit to being antisocial. There is growing evidence that biological and social processes interact in predisposing a person to antisocial behavior (Raine, 2002). The best replicated effect appears to be birth complications interacting with negative home environments in predisposing an individual to adult violence, and this effect particularly characterizes life-course-persistent antisocial behavior (Raine, 2002). Other examples of environmental conditions favoring ASP have recently been recognized. For instance, the relative rate of ASP varies as a function of the nutrition of mothers. From October 1944 to May 1945, the German army blockaded food supplies to the Netherlands, subjecting the western Netherlands first to moderate, then to severe, nutritional deficiency. A follow-up of men who were *in utero* during the famine, and therefore exposed prenatally to severe maternal nutritional deficiency during the first and/or second trimesters of pregnancy, exhibited increased risk for ASP (adjusted odds ratio 2.5; 95% confidence interval 1.5–4.2) (Neugebauer et al., 1999). In other words, when there is a famine during the first and second trimester, there is an increased rate of births of those who will have ASP.

Another possible explanation for the evolutionary role of persons with ASP might be an increase in the variance in mating. Bass, whose exquisite research illuminates the neurobiology of alternative reproductive tactics in singing fish, was asked whether the proportion of the two reproductive male morphs was a constant. He replied that some variation occurs from season to season and certainly within different populations (A. Bass, personal communication, 2003). Asked what the evolutionary advantage might be, he suggested that perhaps it increases the genetic variability available to females in any one nest. Study of the relative variation in the nonassortative matings for antisocial and nonantisocial human males might argue for an evolutionary biological focus other than aggression. In other words, when persons with ASP mate with those without ASP, are their mates more varied than the nonassortative mates of those without ASP? Is one of the evolutionary functions of ASP "stirring the gene pool" or encouraging diversity by deceptive mating?

The worse conditions are, whether famine or abusive parenting, the more likely individuals with ASP are to become part of the population (Raine, 2002). But if utopian environmental conditions, including an absence of violence, were achieved, would CD and ASP disappear? If the evolutionary advantage of CD/ASP is the stirring of the gene pool and avoiding too much homogeneity, then the answer is no.

REFERENCES

Adams J, McClellan J, Douglass D, McCurry C, & Storck M (1995) Sexually inappropriate behaviors in seriously mentally ill children and adolescents. *Child Abuse Negl*, 19:555–568.

Archer J (1988) *The behavioral biology of aggression*. New York: Cambridge University Press.

Ary DV, Duncan TE, Biglan A, Metzler CW, Noell JW, & Smolkowski K (1999) Development of adolescent problem behavior. *J Abnorm Child Psychol*, 27:141–150.

Bagley C, Bolitho F, & Bertrand L (1995) Mental health profiles, suicidal behavior, and community sexual assault in 2,112 Canadian adolescents. *Crisis*, 16:126–131.

Baker R & Bellis M (1995) *Human sperm competition: Copulation, competition and infidelity*. London: Chapman and Hall.

Bardone AM, Moffitt TE, Caspi A, Dickson N, Stanton WR, & Silva PA (1998) Adult physical health outcomes of adolescent girls with conduct disorder, depression, and anxiety. *J Am Acad Child Adolesc Psychiatry*, 37(6):594–601.

Bass A (1992) Dimorphic male brains and alternative reproductive tactics in a vocalizing fish. *Trends Neurosci*, 15:139–145.

Bass AH, Horvath BJ, & Brothers EB (1996) Nonsequential developmental trajectories lead to dimorphic vocal circuitry for males with alternative reproductive tactics. *J Neurobiol*, 30(4):493–504.

Cadoret RJ, Yates WR, Troughton E, Woodworth G, & Stewart MA (1995) Genetic-environmental interaction in the genesis of aggressivity and conduct disorder. *Arch Gen Psychiatry*, 52:916–924.

Cloninger CR & Guze SB (1970) Psychiatric Illness and female criminality: The role of sociopathy and hysteria in antisocial women. *Am J Psychiatry*, 127:303–311.

Compton WM, Cottler LB, Shillington AM, & Price RK (1995) Is antisocial personality disorder associated with increased HIV risk behaviors in cocaine users? *Drug Alcohol Depend*, 37:34–43.

Darwin C (1859) *The origin of species*. New York: Penguin Books, 1968.

Darwin C (1871) *The descent of man*. Amherst, NY: Prometheus Books, 1997.

Darwin C (1872) *The expression of the emotions in man and animals*. Chicago: University of Chicago Press, 1965.

Eisenberg JF (1981) *The mammalian radiations: An analysis of trends in evolution, adaptation and behavior*. Chicago: University of Chicago Press.

Farrington D, Ohlin L, & Wilson JQ (1986) Understanding and controlling crime. New York: Springer-Verlag.

Freud S (1953a) Three essays on sexuality. In J Strachey (Ed.), *Standard edition of the complete psychological works of Sigmund Freud* (Vol. 7). London: Hogarth Press.

Freud S (1953b) Totem and taboo. In J Strachey (Ed.), *Standard edition of the complete psychological works of Sigmund Freud* (Vol. 13). London: Hogarth Press.

Frysztak RJ & Neafsey EJ (1994) The effect of medial frontal cortex lesions on cardiovascular conditioned emotional responses in the rat. *Brain Res*, 643(1–2):181–193.

Galli V, McElroy SL, Soutullo CA, Kizer D, Raute N, Keck PE Jr., & McConville BJ (1999) The psychiatric diagnoses of twenty-two adolescents who have sexually molested other children. *Compr Psychiatry*, 40(2):85–88.

Gill K, Nolimal D, & Crowley TJ (1992) Antisocial personality disorder, HIV risk behavior and retention in methadone maintenance therapy. *Drug Alcohol Dependence*, 30:247–252.

Gladue BA, Boechler M, & McCaul DD (1989) Hormonal response to competition in human males. *Aggressive Behav*, 15:409–422.

Goodwin DW & Guze SB (1979) *Psychiatric diagnosis* (2nd ed.). New York: Oxford University Press.

Guntherschulze J (1979) Studien zur Kenntnis der Regio olfactoria von Wild– und Hausschwein (Sus scrofa L. 1768 un Sus scrofa f.domestica). *Zool anz*, 202:256–279.

Guze SB, Goodwin DW, & Crane JB (1970) A psychiatric study of the wives of convicted felons: An example of assortative mating. *Am J Psychiatry*, 126:1773–1776.

Hamer D & Copeland P (1999) *Living with our genes*. New York: Anchor Books.

Huesmann LR, Eron LD, Lefkowitz MM, & Walder LO (1984) Stability of aggression over time and generations. *Developmental Psychol*, 20:1120–1134.

Hugdahl K (1998) Cortical control of human classical conditioning: Autonomic and positron emission tomography data. *Psychophysiology*, 35(2):170–178.

Jacobs LF, Gaulin SJC, Sherry DF, & Hoffman GE (1990) Evolution of spatial cognition: Sex-specific patterns of spatial behavior predict hippocampal size. *Proc Natl Acad Sci*, 87:6349–6352.

Jerison HJ (1973) *The evolution of brain and intelligence*. New York: Academic Press.

Jerison HJ (1988) The evolutionary biology of intelligence: Afterthoughts. In HJ Jerison & I Jersion (Eds.), *Intelligence and evolutionary biology* (pp. 447–466). New York: Springer-Verlag.

Jessor R & Jessor SL (1977) *Problem behavior and psychosocial development: A longitudinal study of youth*. New York: Academic Press.

King James Version (1976) *The Holy Bible* (Exodus 22:23–25). Nashville, TN: Regency Publishing.

Kessler RC, Berglund PA, Foster CL, Saunders WB, Stang PE, & Walters EE

(1997) Social consequences of psychiatric disorders: II. Teenage parenthood. *Am J Psychiatry*, 154(10):1405–1411.

Knapp R, Marchaterre MA, & Bass AH (1999) Early development of the motor and premotor circuitry of a sexually dimorphic vocal pathway in a teleost fish. *J Neurobiol*, 38(4):475–490.

Kovacs M, Krol RS, & Voti L (1994) Early onset psychopathology and the risk for teenage pregnancy among clinically referred girls. *J Am Acad Child Adolesc Psychiatry*, 33(1):106–113.

Krueger RF, Moffitt TE, Caspi A, Bleske A, & Silva PA (1998) Assortative mating for antisocial behavior: Developmental and methodological implications. *Behav Genet*, 28(3):173–186.

Kruesi MJP, Casanova MF, Mannheim G, & Johnson-Bilder A. (2004) Reduced temporal volume in early onset conduct disorder. *Psychiatry Res*, 132(1): 1–11.

Kruesi MJP, Keller S, & Wagner MW (2003) Neurobiology of aggression. In A Martin, L Scahill, DS Charney, & JF Leckman (Eds.), *Pediatric psychopharmacology: Principles and practice* (pp. 210–223). New York: Oxford University Press.

Kruska D (1980) Domestikationsbedingte Hirngrossenanderungen bei Saugetieren. *Zool Syst Evol-Forsch*, 18:161–195.

Kruska D (1988) Mammalian domestication and its effect on brain structure and behavior. In HJ Jerison & I Jersion (Eds.), *Intelligence and evolutionary biology* (pp. 211–250). New York: Springer-Verlag.

Lahey BB, Applegate B, Barkley RA, Garfinkel B, McBurnett K, Kerdyk L, et al. (1994) DSM-IV field trials for oppositional defiant disorder and conduct disorder in children and adolescents. *Am J Psychiatry*, 151(8):1163–1171.

Leckman JF & Mayes LC (1998) Understanding developmental psychopathology: How useful are evolutionary accounts? *J Am Acad Child Adolesc Psychiatry*, 37:1011–1021.

MacMillan J & Kofoed L (1984) Sociobiology and antisocial personality disorder. *J Nerv Ment Disord*, 172:701–706.

Marmot MG & Shipley MJ (1996) Do socioeconomic differences in mortality persist after retirement? 25 year followup of civil servants from the first Whitehall study. *Br Med J*, 313:1177–1180.

Meyer-Bahlburg HF, Dolezal CL, Wasserman GA, & Jaramillo BM (1999) Prepubertal boys' sexual behavior and behavior problems. *AIDS Educ Prev*, 11(2):174–186.

Neiderhiser JM, Reiss D, Hetherington EM, & Plomin R (1999) Relationships between parenting and adolescent adjustment over time: Genetic and environmental contributions. *Dev Psychol*, 35(3):680–692.

Neugebauer R, Hoek HW, & Susser E (1999) Prenatal exposure to wartime famine and development of antisocial personality disorder in early adulthood. *JAMA*, 282(5):455–462.

Olweus D (1972) Stability of aggressive reaction patterns in males: A review. *Psychol Bull*, 86:852–875.

Patterson GR, DeBaryshe BD, & Ramsey E (1989) A developmental perspective on antisocial behavior. *Am Psychol*, 44(2):329–335.

Quay HC (1979) Classification. In HC Quay & JS Werry (Eds.), *Psychopathological disorders of childhood* (2nd ed.). New York: Wiley.

Raine, A (2002, July). Biosocial studies of antisocial and violent behavior in children and adults: A review. *J Abnorm Child Psychol,* 30(4): 311–326.

Raine A, Lencz T, Bihrle S, LaCasse L, & Colletti P (2000) Reduced prefrontal gray matter volume and reduced autonomic activity in antisocial personality disorder. *Arch Gen Psychiatry,* 57(2):119–127.

Raleigh MJ & McGuire MT (1991) Biodirectional relationships between tryptophan and social behavior in vervet monkeys. *Adv Exp Med Biol,* 294:289–298.

Ramrakha S, Caspi A, Dickson N, Moffitt TE, & Paul C (2000) Psychiatric disorders and risky sexual behaviour in young adulthood: Cross sectional study in birth cohort. *Br Med J,* 29:263–266.

Reiss D, Plomin R, Hetherington EM, Howe GW, Rovine MJ, Tryon A, & Hagan MS (1994) The separate worlds of teenage siblings: An introduction to the study of the nonshared environment and adolescent development. In EM Hetherington & D Reiss (Eds.), *Separate social worlds of siblings: The impact of nonshared environment on development* (pp. 63–109). Hillsdale, NJ: Erlbaum.

Ridley J (1993) *The red queen: Sex and the evolution of human nature.* London: Penguin.

Robins LN (1966) *Deviant children grown up.* Baltimore: Williams & Wilkins.

Robins LN (1978) Sturdy childhood predictors of adult antisocial behavior: Replications from longitudinal studies. *Psychol Med,* 8:611–622.

Robins LN (1985) Epidemiology of antisocial personality. In R Michels, A Cooper, S Guze, et al. (Eds.), *Psychiatry* (Vol. 3, pp. 1–13). Philadelphia: JB Lippincott.

Robins LN, Tipp J, & Przybeck T (1991) Antisocial personality disorder. In LN Robins & DA Regier (Eds.), *Psychiatric disorders in America.* New York: Free Press.

Rolls ET (1999) *The brain and emotion.* Oxford, UK: Oxford University Press.

Rushton JP (1987) Toward a theory of human multiple birthing: Sociobiology and r/K reproductive strategies. *Acta Genet Med Gemellol (Roma),* 36(3):289–296.

Rutter M (1989) Pathways from childhood to adult life. *J Child Psychol Psychiatry,* 30:23–51.

Rutter M, Giller H, & Hagell A (1998) Antisocial behavior by young people. Cambridge, UK: Cambridge University Press.

Rutter M, Silberg J, O'Connor T, et al. (1999) Genetics and child psychiatry: II. Empirical research findings. *J Child Psychol Psychiatry,* 40:19–55.

Scarr S & McCartney K (1983) How people make their own environments: A theory of genotype environmental effects. *Child Dev,* 54:424–435.

Shapiro LE, Leonard CM, Sessions CE, Dewsbury DA, & Insel TR (1991) Comparative neuroanatomy of the sexually dimorphic hypothalamus in monogamous and polygamous voles. *Brain Res*, 541:232–240.

Spalt L (1975) Sexual behavior and affective disorder. *Dis Nerv Sys*, 36:644–647.

Stewart MA, deBlois CS, Meardon J, & Cummings C (1980) Aggressive conduct disorder of children: The clinical picture. *J Nerv Ment Dis*, 168(10):604–610.

Tourian K, Alterman A, Metzger D, Rutherford M, Cacciola JS, & McKay JR (1997) Validiity of three measures of antisociality in predicting HIV risk behaviors in methadone-maintenance patients. *Drug Alcohol Dep*, 47:99–107.

Wigger H (1939) Vergleichende Untersuchungen am Auge von Wild-und Hausschwein unter besonderer Berucksichtigung der Retina. *A Morphol Okol Tiere*, 36:1–20.

Wright R (1995) *The moral animal*. New York: Vintage Books.

CHAPTER 8

Evolutionary Biology of Stress Disorders

PENNY KNAPP

THE EVOLUTIONARY CONTEXT

Frontal cortical and temporal connections are recently evolved, over-lying but not always overriding, primitive cortical circuits. Survival is a prerequisite to reproduction, and avoiding danger, or fighting back, may be necessary in order to survive. The genome has evolved through previous environments of evolutionary adaptedness (EEAs) that were likely various and malign at times (Chisholm, 1993), so behavioral response systems were selected for accordingly (Tooby & Cosmides, 1990, 1992). These older systems allow complex stimuli, related to maintaining homeostasis and allowing survival, to converge upon the amygdala, part of the central nervous system that detects danger and signals for swift protective responses (Damasio, 1994). The fuse to ignite reflex, cardiopulmonary, and muscle reaction to sudden danger is the allostatic or stress response system, mediated by corticosteriods and neurotransmitters, especially catecholamines.

For a social animal, danger may come from, or be communicated by, other animals. Such signal information is linked in to the emergency response system, through extended connections of the amygdala with projections to the cortex, where activation of dendritic elaborations is experienced as conscious engagement in emotionally charged events (LeDoux, 1994; Rogan & LeDoux, 1996). Parallel to the more recently evolved circuits, the activation of primitive circuits infuses events between and around us with emotional intensity and meaning. In a social group, the large-brained primate is capable of cooperation, problem solving, and planning. More graduated and subtler analytical brain circuits are built out from the primitive networks iteratively (Kinney et al., 1988), through experience that includes a series of transactions. Beginning in infancy, these transactions occur between the infant and his or her caregiver(s) in individually particular ways (Davidson & Fox, 1988), optimally in a relationship buffered from stress (Coplan et al., 1996). However, reproduction is the ultimate evolutionary goal, and alternative parenting strategies may develop in alternative EEAs (Belsky et al., 1984, 1991; Chisholm, 1996). Building in the "civilized," gratification-delaying, empathetic, problem-solving circuits is a long process with a fragile product. Stress, particularly interpersonal stress, may activate the archaic response patterns (Goerner, 1995; LeDoux, 1996; Schore, 1997). The inner lizard crouches within the thinking human.

Stress, for the immature animal, includes neglect. Mechanisms by which neglect stresses the infant are described in Chapter 3. Briefly, the balance between experiences, such as hunger, that painfully overstimulate him, and experiences of being fed or soothed, that restore him to a calm state is frequently absent. The infant's developing brain adapts to this by constructing patterns of regulation that are poorly modulated, so he may cry unappeased until he exhausts himself or withdraws into a conserving state of diminished responsiveness.

The stress response system has evolved to effect the survival of animals capable, under fire of stress, of soldering vital memories about good or terrifying events, by means of corticosteroid activation of the network between the hippocampus and the amygdala. This process constructs the earliest maps of emotional terrains through activation of biogenic aminergic systems that regulate the growth and tonus of the limbic system and its frontotemporal cortical connections. Those maps underlie the later-developing, more cognitive, analytical, and modulated routes for information processing. However, they are never buried far below the surface; stress impairs prefrontal cortical function (Arnstein, 1999), and the primal capacity to short-circuit the routes to higher cortical domains in favor of primally life-saving faster reflexive processing through the thalmus and amygdala persists (LeDoux, 1996, pp. 163–165).

RESILIENCE: EARLY AFFECTS AND LOVE MAPS

All the contingent and noncontingent actions of his or her care-giver(s) are experiences for the infant. The infant's brain, in a growth boom, lays down neuronal and dendritic connections from these ex-periences, spending neuronal materials judiciously (Cherniak, 1995), embedding many subsystems within cortical maps (Krubitizer, 1995), and deploying neurotransmitters flexibly. Selective expression of the infant's genes, catalysts of his or her new learning, and the building, remodeling, and organization of his or her brain, are modulated by the infant's affective states.

Underlying the rich affective communications between parent and offspring are the communications necessary for survival. To sur-vive danger and form affiliations, social animals must accurately rec-ognize emotion and must be able to communicate emotion. The amygdala, integral to the danger-detecting archaic neural system, re-ceives complex stimuli related to homeostatic status and environ-mental hazard and signals rapid protective responses, short-circuiting slower cortical pathways (Damasio, 1994). The intense and instanta-neous signals, which we label "emotions," arise in the amygdala (LeDoux, 1994; Rodrigues et al., 2004; Rogan & LeDoux, 1996) and are relayed on to the adjacent hippocampus, catalyzing memory encoding. The amygdala's role in decoding facial expression is seen on fMRI (functional magnetic resonance imagery) in even young hu-mans (Baird et al., 1999) and is independent of age and gender.

Brain self-organization is an ongoing process. Elaboration and differentiation of cortical circuits, and, after the second year, the de-velopment of language, will build a neuronal matrix that can be acti-vated flexibly for alternative responses to experiences. The develop-ment in the first year, however, lays down at least two parallel and overlapping systems of emotional regulation (LeDoux, 1992, 1994; Schore, 1997) that counterbalance each other. They are variously termed excitatory and inhibitory, or cortical and subcortical systems. The first attachment(s) set the first regulatory balances of delight versus despair, affiliation versus alienation, resiliency (Werner, 1995) versus vulnerability (Wang & Pitts, 1994). This charts a course toward trusting intimacy or toward apprehensive avoidance of others, or uncertain voyages in the territories between, guided by changing love maps. "Love maps" is a term for the familiar patterns of response constructed in the course of intimate relationships. The earliest intimate relationship is that between the infant and his or her mother.

Self-regulation in childhood and adulthood can now begin to be examined with the techniques of neuroimaging (Posner & Rothbart, 2000; Shulman, 2001). Smaller hippocampal volume may not be predictive of posttraumatic stress disorder (PTSD) (Bonne et al., 2001) but may be observed in individuals with early or prolonged PTSD (e.g. Bremner et al 1997), although, in a small sample of children studied longitudinally, it was not associated with PTSD.

Clinically, it is observed that attachment is protective against the extremes of stress response. Orphans who had experienced 8 or more months of institutional rearing had higher salivary cortisol than those with shorter stays in institutions or matched controls (Gunnar & Chilsholm, 1991). Secure attachment relationships are associated with moderated cortisol responses to a novel situation of 18-month-old children who are behaviorally inhibited (Gunnar et al., 1996). Maladaptive parental behavior has been shown to be associated with psychiatric disorders in children (Johnson et al., 2001), and this effect is increased by early childbearing and low maternal educational level (Nagin & Tremblay, 2001) and by maternal depression (Dawson et al., 1999). Parental buffering of trauma, and the influence of interpersonal stabilization or destabilization of its effects in the manifestations of traumatic stress, remain active areas of study (Volkmar, 2001).

ALTERNATIVE ORGANIZATIONS OF STRESS MODULATION: CLINICAL SYNDROMES

Excessive stress and early trauma are known to influence the calibration of the homeostatic process and to bring about enduring resets of neurobiological regulatory systems (Emde, 1989; Glod & Teicher, 1996; Lieberman & Zeanah, 1995; Main, 2000; Pine et al., 1998). Transient changes in infant noradrenaline levels may permanently reset the equilibration point of the system (Higley et al., 1991; Post & Weiss, 1997). Childhood PTSD produces changes that result in symptoms, particularly affective symptoms and anxiety dysregulation, that may persist into adulthood (Terr, 1991). Girls may be more vulnerable than boys (Hubbard et al., 1995). Maltreated children with PTSD are likelier to have symptoms that persist (Famularo et al., 1996a) and that may be consistent with ADHD, other anxiety disorders, psychotic symptoms, suicidal ideation, and mood symptoms (Famularo et al., 1996b). Symptoms of avoidance and numbing, present long after a traumatic event, may be elicited in a dynamic interpersonal interview but may not be reported on structured clinical interviews (Honig et al., 1999). This is consistent with the findings implicating, in response to trauma, alteration in brain regions that regulate emotion and stress, not only those regulating cognitive processing of verbal information (Damasio, 1994). Dissociative symptoms, in particular, have been difficult to quantify or predict (Bremner, 1999), and the probabilities of developing dissociative symptoms versus intrusive symptoms in response to severe stress have eluded diagnostic prediction. That both could arise from the same insult is understandable if we recall that the coriticosteroid activation elicited by stress leads, in a nonlinear fashion, to direct, indirect, and compensatory events in the brain. Bremner (1999) proposes a new category of trauma spectrum disorders that would allow incorporating seemingly conflicting findings. This would allow the descriptive system to be less rigid, but would still not explain how homeostatic processes, to which our evolution has made us heirs, have brought about the changes in self-regulation that are classified as psychiatric symptoms.

Genes constrain development, but in a sometimes negotiable way, and the genetic predispostion to dissociation or other posttraumatic stress reactions has not been clarified. Dramatic developmental deviation may also result from early stress that alters mitochondrial function (Kimberg et al., 1968), brain energy metabolism, and corticosteroid receptor settings (Bryan 1990) through hyperactivation of excitotoxic N-methyl-D-aspartate (NMDA)–sensitive glutamate receptors, synapse elimination, and neurotoxicity (Benes et al., 1994). The immature host of such processes, especially if his or her interpersonal experiences are inconsistent and unpredictable, is the child with a disorganized–disoriented attachment (Main & Solomon, 1986) or PTSD (Cicchetti & Toth, 1995). To a treacherous interpersonal environment, the developing child adapts with increased cortisol production, parasympathetic vagal-associated dissociation, or protracted hyperarousal and hypoarousal (Perry et al., 1995). The child's circadian rhythms may be disrupted, his or her mood expression may appear unmodulated (Glod & Teicher, 1996), and his or her aggression and activity levels may be higher. The child is likely to have a negative internal representation of him- or herself and negative expectations of others. The child's interactions will be more controlling and less responsive (Toth et al., 1997).

Infants whose mothers, because of depression, cannot provide contingent responses and optimal levels of stimulation, suffer compromised experience-expectant social learning (Field, 1995). They also manifest atypical frontal EEG patterns—reduced activity over the left frontal scalp region, as compared with infants of nondepressed mothers, not associated with affective behavior during the structured conditions of recording (Dawson et al., 1999). This is consistent with theoretical and experimental links of the left frontal region with approach behaviors and the right frontal region with withdrawal behaviors (Davidson et al., 1990). As toddlers, the same children show less coordinated interactions, fewer positive and more hostile or aggressive behaviors, and apparent difficulty with self-organization (Dawson et al., 1999).

The observations of neuroanatomic change must be interpreted in a developmental context. Neurophysiological response algorithms, as social learning, are self-perpetuating. Stressed children may continue to generate their own stress in a transactional fashion with their parents and peers (Rudolph et al., 2000).

POSTTRAUMATIC STRESS DISORDER

When the stress response system is maximally activated, a variable constellation of responses is triggered. The patterns of response are generally grouped as arousal, dissociative, or mixed patterns. The manifestations—biological, emotional, and behavioral—recognized as symptoms, are termed acute stress disorder or PTSD. Symptoms may be prolific and pleiomorphic (Pelcovitz & Kaplan, 1996; Pfefferbaum, 1997). Improved understanding of their neurobiological underpinnings is possible with new neuroimaging techniques (e.g., Pitman et al., 2001). They may often appear as or with learned or burned-in behavioral and emotional response patterns that meet diagnostic criteria for other DSM-IV (American Psychiatric Association, 1994) diagnoses. Attention-deficit/hyperactivity disorder, conduct disorder, anxiety disorder, and bipolar affective disorder (Hubbard et al., 1995) are frequently comorbidly diagnosed with PTSD and with each other (Weller et al., 1995). The arousal symptoms of PTSD—sleep difficulties, hypervigilance, irritability, and poor concentration—are "externalizing" symptoms. The dissociative symptoms of the child with PTSD, as well as anxiety, mistrust, avoidance, futurelessness, and depression, are "internalizing" symptoms. The child's adaptive coping with the trauma may take the form of behaviors that are perceived as symptoms (Terr, 1981). Diagnostic schemes such as DSM-IV are of value in describing symptoms that have stability over time (Achenbach, 1991; Lavigne et al., 1998a; Lavigne et al., 1998b; Lucas et al., 2001). However, a symptom-listing diagnostic scheme, which has serious limitations in describing adult "psychopathology," may be barely meaningful at all in understanding symptoms in the developing child. Moreover, the DSM-IV treats phenomena as categorical that may be on a continuum (Jensen, 1995; Jensen et al., 1999; Levy et al., 1997), while minimizing consideration of the particular contexts in which those phenomena may become more pronounced. Semistructured interviews, in the hands of trained clinicians (Geller et al., 2001), better combine qualitative and specific clinical observations.

Conservative estimates of children in the United States exposed to trauma per year number 4 million (e.g., Finkelhor & Dziuba-Leatherman, 1994; Perry & Pate, 1994). Many have emotional or behavioral sequelae (Brown et al., 1999). Just as the vulnerability of a child or adolescent varies, so does the degree of trauma. Thus, one cannot expect a certain level of posttraumatic stress to be a linear function of the amount of stress the individual experienced.

Trauma suffered by children and adolescents may be grouped at three general levels: harm to the child (e.g., neglect, witnessing domestic violence), harm inflicted by a bigger person or in the family (e.g., nonaccidental trauma, sexual abuse, intrafamilial abuse), and harm in the community (Knapp et al., 2001), as shown in Table 8.1. The table offers a general framework for determining how a trauma may harm a child or adolescent. This framework is theoretical. Of course, human suffering does not always follow theoretical organizations. For example, traumatized children are also frequently ne-

TABLE 8.1. Planning Treatment for the Abused Child

Level where the abuse occurred	Where is the harm?	What treatment might apply to this level?
Harm to the child • Neglect • Domestic violence • Witnessing (e.g., fatal family) violence	In the brain, body memories, distorted cognitions, sensitized neurobiology	*Treatment of the child* • Medications • Biofeedback, stress reduction/management • Psychotherapy, cognitive-behavioral therapy
Harm between the child and another person • Sexual abuse • Neglect • Physical, nonaccidental • Intrafamilial (incest)	In the relationship between the child and his or her caregivers or a perpetrator	*Treatment of the child in the child's relationship(s)* • Cognitive-behavioral therapy • Parent–child interaction therapy (if parent involved) • Behavior management • Family therapy • Group therapy
Harm in the community • Community violence • Aggravating factors (e.g., cultural shame or poverty)	In the context of the child and caregiver and their community	*Intervention at the level of the family/community* • Family therapy • Group therapy • Peer therapy

glected (e.g., National Research Council, 1993; Pynoos et al., 1996). Particularly in cases of in-home abuse, the presence of neglect and its effects should be considered when assessing the mental health needs of a traumatized child. Many children suffer more than one kind of trauma and are harmed in several ways, so the effect of a particular trauma may be magnified. A child may be more vulnerable to one trauma because of preceding harm, and children who are traumatized may experience trauma at more than one level. The implication for treatment planning is that treatment may also need to be addressed on more than one level. For example, a child may need both stress reduction and behavioral management or family therapy.

A relationship between distress symptoms and exposure to violence has been demonstrated, and it has been shown that even after removal to foster care, children may continue to be exposed to community violence (Stein et al., 2001). Violence exposure has been shown to be associated with psychological trauma, suicidal risk, and violent behavior (Flannery et al., 2001). Children's reactions to stress, like all their learning in interpersonal contexts, is best understood in a transactional model (Rutter et al., 1997). The adapting individual continuously negotiates a dynamic balance between developmental maturation, optimum stimulus seeking, and stress. Resilience is constructed among moderating and mediating influences. These factors must be considered and understood as well as possible before planning treatment.

TREATMENT

Recent studies of evidence-based treatment methods with roots in cognitive, social learning, and behavioral treatment models have begun to demonstrate the usefulness of these methods in treating child victims of trauma. Therapies founded on psychodynamic theory have not been much represented in the recent empirical research because of greater methodological obstacles. The growing availability of better biological measures, including, for example, functional magnetic resonance imaging (fMRI) as an assessment tool, shows great promise for examining changes resulting from therapy. For example, emotional and cognitive activation elicits different patterns of regional metabolic change in brain activity in patients with PTSD than in persons without PTSD (Shin et al., 2001). Symptom provocation elicited by script-driven imagery also creates observed changes in regional brain activity (Rauch et al., 1996). A continuum of treatment methods, applied appropriately and competently, may produce positive outcomes for traumatized children. At the optimum end of the continuum are treatments based on substantial empirical evidence (such as well-controlled double-blind trials) and/or overwhelming clinical consensus, or legal and regulatory requirements. Next most desirable are treatments that are based on empirical evidence (such as case series and open trials) and/or strong clinical consensus. Some treatment options are practices that are acceptable, but for which there may be insufficient empirical evidence to support recommending them as best practices or clinical standards, although in particular cases they may be the best approach. For a recent review, see Knapp and colleagues (2001).

Classifying risk factors into proxy, overlapping, and independent risk factors, and factors that are mediating and moderating may point to ways to identify children at particular risk and may guide the context and strategies for intervention (Kraemer et al., 2001). A first order of business is to protect the child from further harm. Treatment should be relevant to both the trauma and the child's adaptation to it. Generally, the earlier in development the trauma or neglect has occurred, the more primitive the brain systems whose organization may have been jeopardized by the stress. Thus, to plan treatment for a child, it is crucial to get a developmental history that explores the timing of the stress and the available attachment support during that stage of development.

To plan treatment that allows recovery and resumption of growth, it may be necessary to alter abnormal response patterns at any or all of the following levels. If disruption of regulation has occurred at the level of the midbrain and/or diencephalon, a treatment goal will be to restore regularity, rest, stability of diet, sleep, and daily schedule. If disruption has been in regulation involving the limbic system, a treatment goal will be to help the child label but contain emotions, to foster affective constancy, and to support attachment. To restore self-organization at the cortical level, treatment goals are for the child to be able to talk about feelings, not only act in response to them, and to strengthen top-down restructuring of experiences. Treatment goals will be to move the child's cognitive style from reflexive/reactive through emotional, to concrete, to abstract thought. As treatment progresses, the child's internal state will move from predominantly a fear/alarm state, through tolerable arousal to equinimity. This will allow his or her attentional patterns to move from inattention/dissociation through compliance/imitation and/or avoidance to alert calm (Perry et al., 1995).

For each type of trauma, treatment planning will be predicated on defining the trauma, the child's experience, the child's coping/defense/processing of the experience, context factors conditions for treatment, challenges to treatment, and possibly effective treatment modalities (Knapp et al., 2001). The level of treatment, derived from the individual's biological response to the community processing of the trauma, will define the possibilities for the type of treatment to be chosen. Table 8.2 shows the theoretical relationships of treatment models to types of specific treatments and their proposed actions.

Treatment approaches selected will be aimed at symptom abatement, for example, management and reduction of avoidance symptoms, or expression and management of emotions, especially those

TABLE 8.2. Models of Treatment, Treatment Types, and Possible Effects

Theoretical model	Treatment type	How treatment might work
Individual: Biological	• Medications • Biofeedback • Stress management	Treatments proposed to re-regulate neurobiological responses that have been altered by the stress, to a more normal pattern.
Individual: Psychological	• Psychotherapy: play therapy, cognitive-behavioral therapy, cognitive coping triangle • Exposure techniques • Correcting inaccurate attributions	Treatments proposed to teach the child, cognitively and/or through a learned new relationship with a trustable therapist, to master the trauma and to respond differently to new life experiences.
Interpersonal: Family relationships	• Parent–child interaction or family therapy • Group or peer therapy	Treatments proposed to change the patterns of family and interpersonal relationships, so that the child is furnished with new experiences that will correct the patterns established by the earlier traumatic experiences.
Psychosocial: Ecological	Approaches to a group of individuals, children, and parents who have been traumatized	Similar to the three treatment approaches above, but the intervention addresses the community context as well as interpersonal relationships within the group.

related to traumatic events, or correction of cognitive distortions, or behavior containment and self-regulation. This will pull the child from the whirlpool of overactivated stress responses. However, treatment can also bring the child forward, moving him or her into a developmentally appropriate current, one in which the child's relationships are rewarding, his or her cognitive activities are optimally stimulating, and his or her emotions are deep but modulated. When this occurs, the adaptive mechanisms selected by evolution will again work in the child's favor, and not against the child.

REFERENCES

Achenbach TM (1991) *Manual for the Child Behavior Checklist 4/18 and 1991 profile.* Burlington: University of Vermont, Department of Psychiatry.

Allmann JM (1998) *Evolving brains.* New York: W.H. Freeman (Scientific American).

American Psychiatric Association (1994) *Diagnostic and statistical manual of mental disorders* (4th ed.). Washington DC: Author.

Arnstein AFT (1999) Development of the cerebral cortex: XIV. Stress impairs prefrontal cortical function. *J Am Acad Child Adolesc Psychiatry,* 38(2):220–222.

Baird AA, Gruber SA, Fein DA, Maas LC, Stengard RJ, Renshaw PF, Cohen BM, & Yurgelun-Todd DA (1999) Functional magnetic resonance imaging of facial affect recognition in children and adolescents. *J Am Acad Child Adolesc Psychiatry,* 38(2):195–199.

Beauchaine R (2001) Vagal tone, development, and Gray's motivational theory: Toward an integrated model of autonomic nervous system functioning in psychopathology. *Dev Psychopathology,* 13:183–214.

Beebe B & Lachmann FM (1988) Mother–infant mutual influence and precursors of psychic structure. In A. Goldberg (Ed.), *Progress in self psychology* (Vol. 3, p. 325). Hillsdale, NJ: Analytic Press.

Belsky J, Rovine M, & Taylor DG (1984) The Pennsylvania Infant and Family Development Project. III: The origins of individual differences in infant–mother attachment: Maternal and infant contributions. *Child Dev,* 55:718–728.

Belsky J, Steinberg L, & Draper P (1991) Childhood experience, interpersonal development, and reproductive strategy: An evolutionary theory of socialization. *Child Dev,* 62:1224–1231.

Bremner JD (1999) Acute and chronic responses to psychological trauma: Where do we go from here? *Am J Psychiatry* 156:349–351.

Bremner JD, Randall PR, Vermetten E, Staib L, Bronen RA, Mazure C, Capelli S, McCarthy G, Innis RG, & Charney DS (1997) MRI-based measurement of hippocampal volume in posttraumatic stress disorder related to childhood physical and sexual abuse: A preliminary report. *Biol Psychiatry,* 41:23–32.

Benes FM, Turtle M, Khan Y, & Farol P (1994) Myelination of a key relay zone in the hippocampal formation occurs in the human brain during childhood, adolescence, and adulthood. *Arch Gen Psychiatry,* 51(6):477–484.

Bonne O, Brandes D, Gilboa A, Gomori JM, Shenton ME, Pitman RK, & Shalev AY (2001) Longitudinal MRI study of hippocampal volume in trauma survivors with PTSD. *Am J Psychiatry,* 158(8):1248–1251.

Brown J, Cohen P, Johnson JG, & Smailes EM (1999). Child abuse and neglect: Specificity of effects on adolescent and young adult depression and suicidality. *J Am Acad Child Adolesc Psychiatry* 38:1490–1496.

Bryan RM Jr. (1990) Cerebral blood flow and energy metabolism during stress. *Am J Physiol* 259:H269–H280.

Cherniak C (1995) Neural component placement. *Trends Neurosci*, 18:522–527.

Chisholm JS (1993) Death, hope, and sex: Life-history theory and the development of reproductive strategies. *Curr Anthropol*, 34:1–24.

Chisholm JS (1996) The evolutionary ecology of attachment organization. *Hum Nature*, 7:1–38.

Cicchetti D & Toth SL (1995) A developmental psychopathology perspective on child abuse and neglect. *J Am Acad Child Adolesc Psychiatry*, 34: 541–565.

Coplan JD, Andrews MW, Rosenblum LA, Owens MJ, Friedman S, Gorman JM, & Nemeroff CB (1996) Persistent elevations of cerebrospinal fluid concentrations of corticotropin-relasing factor in adult nonhuman primates exposed to early-life stressors: Implications for the pathophysiology of mood and anxiety disorders. *Proc Nat Acad Sci U.S.A.*, 93: 1619–1623.

Courchesne E, Chisum H, & Townsend J (1994) Neural activity-dependent brain changes in development: Implications for psychopathology: Neural plasticity, sensitive periods and psychopathology [Special issue]. *Dev Psychopathology*, 6:697–722.

Damasio AR (1994) *Descartes' error: Emotion, reason and the human brain.* New York: Grosset/Putnam.

Davidson RJ, Ekman P, Saron C, Senulis R, & Friesen WV (1990) Approach–withdrawal and cerebral asymmetry: Emotional expression and brain physiology: I. *J Pers Soc Psychol*, 58:330–341.

Davidson RJ & Fox NA (1988) Cerebral asymmetry and emotion: Development and individual differences. In DL Molfese & SJ Segalowitz (Eds.), *Brain lateralization in children: Developmental implications* (pp. 191–206). New York: Guilford Press.

Dawson G (1994) Frontal electroencephalographic correlates of individual differences in emotion expression in infants: A brain systems perspective on emotion. In NA Fox (Ed.), *The development of emotion regulation: Biological and behavioral considerations. Monogr Soc Res Child Dev*, 65(2–3, Serial No. 240):135–151.

Dawson G, Frey K, Panagiotides H, Osterling J, & Hessl D (1997) Infants of depressed mothers exhibit atypical frontal brain activity: A replication and extension of previous findings. *J Child Psychol Psychiatry*, 38:179–186.

Dawson G, Frey K, Self J, Panagiotides H, Hessle D, Yamada E, & Rinaldi J (1999) Frontal electrical brain activity in infants of depressed mothers: Relation of variations in infant behavior. *Dev Psychopathology*, 11:589–605.

Dawson G, Hessl D, & Frey K (1994) Social influences of early developing biological and behavioral systems related to risk for affective disorder: Neural plasticity, sensitive periods and psychopathology. [Special issue]. *Dev Psychopathology*, 6:759–779.

Emde RN (1989) The infant's relationship experience: Developmental and affective aspects. In A Sameroff & RM Emde (Eds.), *Relationship disturbances in early childhood: A developmental approach* (pp. 33–51). New York: Basic Books.

Famularo R, Fenton T, Augustyn M, & Zuckerman B (1996) Persistence of pediatric post traumatic stress disorder after 2 years. *Child Abuse Negl*, 20(12):1245–1248.

Famularo R, Fenton T, Kinscherff R, & Augustyn M. (1996) Psychiatric comorbidity in childhood post traumatic stress disorder. *Child Abuse Negl*, 20(10):953–961.

Field T (1995) Infants of depressed mothers. *Infant Behav Dev*, 18:1–13.

Finkelhor D & Dziuba-Leatherman J (1994) Children as victims of violence: A national survey. *Pediatrics*, 94:413–420.

Flannery DJ, Singer MI, & Wester K (2001) Violence exposure, psychological trauma, and suicide risk in a community sample of dangerously violent adolescents. *J Am Acad Child Adolesc Psychiatry*, 40(4):435–442.

Fox NA, Schmidt LA, Calkins SD, Rubin KH, & Coplan RJ (1996) The role of frontal activation in the regulation and dysregulation of social behavior during the preschool years. *Dev Psychopathology*, 8:89–102.

Geller B, Zimerman B, Williams M, Bolhofner K, Craney JL, DelBello M, & Soutullo C (2001) Reliability of the Washington University in St. Louis Kiddie Schedule for Affective Disorders and Chisophrenia (WASH-U-KSADS) Mania and Rapid Cycling Sections. *JAACAP*, 40(4):450–455).

Glod CA & Teicher MH (1996) Relationship between early abuse, post-traumatic stress disorder and activity levels in prepubertal children. *J Am Acad Child Adolesc Psychiatry*, 35(10):1384–1393.

Goerner S (1995) Chaos, evolution and deep ecology. In R Robertson & A Combs (Eds.), *Chaos theory in pychology and the life sciences* (pp. 17–38). Mahwah, NJ: Erlbaum.

Gorski RA (1999) Development of the cerebral cortex: XV. Sexual differentiation of the central nervous system. *Am Acad Child Adolesc Psychiatry*, 38 (3):344–346.

Greenough WT, Black JE, & Wallace CS (1987) Experience and brain development. *Child Dev*, 58:539–559.

Gunnar MR, Broderson L, Nachimias M, Buss K, & Rigatuso J (1996) Stress reactivity and attachment security. *Dev Psycho*, 29:191–204.

Gunnar MR & Chisholm KC (1991, April) *Effects of early institutional rearing and attachment quality on salivary cortisol levels in adopted Romanian children*. Poster session presented at the biennial meeting of the Society for Research in Child Development, Albuquerque, NM.

Higley JD, Suomi SJ, & Linnoila M (1991) CSF monoamine metabolite concentrations vary according to age, rearing and sex, and are influenced by the stressor of social separation in rhesus monkeys. *Psychopharmacology*, 103:551–556.

Honig RG, Grace MC, Lindy JD, Newman CJ, & Titchener JL (1999) Assessing long-term effects of trauma: diagnosing symptoms of avoidance and numbing. *Am J Psychiatry*, 156(3):483–485.

Hubbard, J, Realmuto GM, Northwoood AK, & Masten AS (1995) Comorbidity of psychiatric diagnoses with posttraumatic stress disorder in survivors of chldhood trauma. *J Am Acad Child Adolesc Psychiatry*, 34:1167–1173.

Insel TR & Hulihan TJ 1995 A gender specific mechanism for pair bonding: Oxytocin and partner preference formation in monogamous voles. *Behav Neurosci*, 109(4):782–789.

Insel TR, Preston S, & Winslow JT 1995 Mating in the monogamous male: Behavioral consequences. Physiol Behav, 57(4):615–627.

Jacobsen L & Sapolsky R (1991) The role of the hippocampus in the feedback regulation of the hypothalamic–pituitary–adrenocortical axis. *Endochrinology Rev*, 12:118–134.

Jensen PS (1995) Scales versus categories? Never play against a stacked deck. *J Am Acad Child Adolesc Psychiatry*, 34:485–487.

Jensen PS, Brooks-Gunn J, & Graber JA (1999) Dimensional scales and diagnostic categories: Constructing crosswalks for child psychopathology assessments. *J Am Acad Child Adolesc Psychiatry*, 34:485–487.

Johnson JG, Cohen P, Casen S, Smailes E, & Brook JS (2001) Association of maldaptive parental behavior with psychiatric disorder among parents and their offspring. *Arch Gen Psychiatry*, 58:453–460.

Kaufer D, Friedman A, & Soreq H (1999) The vicious circle of stress and anticholinesterase response. *Neuroscientist*, 5(3):173–183.

Kimberg DV, Loud AV, & Wiener A (1968) Cortisone-induced alterations in mitochondrial function and structure. *J Cell Biol*, 37:63–67.

Kinney HC, Brody BA, Kloman AS, & Gilles FH (1988) Sequence of central nervous system myelination in human infancy: II. Patterns of myelination in autopsied infants. *J Neuropathol Exp Neurol*, 47:217–234.

Knapp PK, Urquiza A, Kent J, & Winterstein M. (2001) Treatment of child crime victims. In M Winterstein & SR Scribner (Eds.), *Mental health care for child crime victims: Standards of care task force guidelines* (pp. 5-1–5-20). Sacramento: California Victim Compensation and Government Claims Board Victims of Crime Program.

Kraemer HC, Stice E, Kazdin A, Offord D, & Kupfer D (2001). How do risk factors work together? Mediators, moderators and independent overlapping and proxy risk factors. *Am J Psychiatry*, 158(6):848–856.

Krubitzer L (1995) The organization of neocortex in mammals: are species differences really so different? *Trends Neurosci*, 18:408–417.

Lavigne JV, Arend R, Rosenbaum D, Binns JH, Chrisoffel K, & Gibbons RD

(1998a) Psychiatric disorders with onset in preschool years: I. Stability of diagnosis. *J Am Acad Child Adolesc Psychiatry*, 37(12):1246–1254.

Lavigne JV, Binns JH, Arend R, Rosenbaum D, Chrisoffel K, Hayford JR, & Gibbons RD (1998b) Psychopathology and health care use among preschool children: A restrospective analysis. *J Am Acad Child Adolesc Psychiatry*, 37(3):262–270.

LeDoux JE (1994) Emotion, memory and the brain. *Sci Am*, 270:50–57.

LeDoux JE (1996) *The emotional brain*. New York: Simon & Schuster.

Levy F, Hay DA, McStephen M, Wood C, & Waldman I (1997) Attention-deficit hyperactivity disorder: A category or a continuum? Genetic analysis of a large-scale twin study. *J Am Acad Child Adolesc Psychiatry*, 36(6):737–744.

Lieberman AF & Zeanah CH (1995) Disorders of attachment in infancy. *Child Adolesc Psychiatric Clin North Am*, 4(3):571–587.

Lucas CP, Zhang H, Fisher PW, Shaffer D, Regier DA, Narrow WE, Bourdon K, Lahey B, & Friman P (2001) The DISC predictive scales (DPS) efficiently screening for diagnoses. *JAACAP*, 40(4):443–449.

Main M (2000) The organized categories of infant, child, and adult attachment: flexible vs. inflexible attention under attachment-related stress. *J Am Psychoanal Assoc*, 48(4):1055–1096.

Main M & Solomon J (1986) Discovery of an insecure-disorganized/disoriented attachment pattern. In TB Brazelton & M W Yogman (Eds.), *Affective development in infancy*. Norwood, NJ: Ablex.

Nagin DS & Tremblay RE (2001) Parental and early childhood predictors of persistent physical aggression in boys from kindergarten to high school. *Arch Gen Psychiatry*, 58:389–394.

National Research Council (1993) *Understanding child abuse and neglect*. Washington, DC: National Academy Press.

Newcomer JW, Selke GS, Melson AK, Hershey T, Craft S, Richards K, & Alderson AL (1999) Decreased memory performance in healthy humans induced by stress-level cortisol treatment. *Arch Gen Psychiatry*, 56:527–553.

Novelli A, Reilly JA, Lysko, PG, & Henneberry RC (1988) Glutamate becomes neurotoxic via the N-methyl-D-aspartate receptor when intracellular energy levels are reduced. *Brain Res*, 451:205–212.

Perry BD & Pate JE (1994) Neurodevelopment and the psychobiological roots of post-traumatic stress disorders. In LF Koziol & CE Stout (Eds.), *The neuropsychology of mental disorders. A practical guide*. Springfield, IL: Thomas.

Perry DB, Pollard RA, Blakley TL, Maker WL, & Vigilante D (1995) Childhood trauma: The neurobiology of adaptation and "use-dependent" development of the brain: How states become traits. *Infant Ment Health*, 16:271–291.

Pelcovitz D & Kaplan S (1996) Post traumatic stress disorder in children and adolescents. *Child Adolesc Psychiatric Clin North Am*, 5(5):449–469.

Pfefferbaum B (1997) Posttraumatic stress disorder in children: A review of the past 10 years. *J Am Acad Child Adolesc Psychiatry*, 36(11):1503–1511.

Pine D, Cohen P, Gurley D, Brook J, & Ma Y (1998) The risk for early-adulthood anxiety and depressive disorders in adolescents with anxiety and depressive disorders. *Arch Gen Psychiatry*, 55:56–64.

Pitman RK, Shin LM, & Rauch SL (2001) Investigating the pathogenesis of posttraumatic stress disorder with neuroimaging. *J Clin Psychiatry*, 62(Suppl 17):47–54.

Porges SW (1990) Vagal tone: An autonomic mediator of affect. In J Garber & K Dodge (Eds.), *The development of emotion regulation and dysregulation* (pp. 111–128). New York: Cambridge University Press.

Porges SW (1995) Orienting in a defensive world: Mammalian modifications of our evolutionary heritage: A polyvagal theory. *Psychophysiology*, 32:301–318.

Porges SW, Doussard-Roosevelt JA, & Maiti AK (1994) Vagal tone and the physiological regulation of emotion. *Monog Soc Res Child Dev*, 59:167–186.

Posner MI & Rothbart MK (2000) Develolping mechanisms of self-regulation. *Dev Psychopathology*, 12:427–441.

Post RM & Weiss SRB (1997): Emergent properties of neural systems: How focal molecular neurobiological alterations can affect behavior. *Dev Psychopathology*, 9(4):907–930.

Purves D & LaMantia AS (1990) Construction of modular circuits in the mammalian brain. *Cold Spring Harbor Sym Quant Biol*, 55:445–452.

Pynoos RS, Steinberg AM, & Goenjian A (1996) Traumatic stress in childhood and adolescence: Recent developments and current controversies. In BA van der Kolk, AC McFarlane, CL Weisaeth (Eds.), *Traumatic stress: The effects of overwhelming experience on mind, body, and society* (pp. 331–358). New York: Guilford Press.

Rauch SL, van der Kolk BA, Fisler RE, Alpert NM, Orr SP, Savage CR, Fischman AJ, Jenicke MA, & Pitman RK (1996) A symptom provocation study of posttraumatic stress disorder using positron emission tomography and script-driven imagery. *Arch Gen Psychiatry*, 53:380–387.

Rogan MT & LeDoux JE (1996) Emotion: Systems, cells, synaptic plasticity. *Cell*, 85:469–475.

Rubin KH, Hastings P, Chen X, Stewart S, & McNichol K (1998) Intrapersonal and maternal correlates of aggression, conflict and externalizing problems in toddlers. *Child Dev*, 69(6):1614–1629.

Rudolph KD, Hammen C, Burge D, Lindberg N, Herzberg D, & Daley SE (2000) Toward an interpersonal life-stress model of depression: The developmental context of stress generation. *Dev Psychopathology*, 12:215–234.

Rutter M, Dunn J, Plomin R, Simonoff E, Pickles A, Maughan B, Ormel J, Meyer J, & Eaves L (1997) Integrating nature and nurture: Implications of person–environment correlations and interactions for developmental psychopathology. *Dev Psychopathology*, 9:335–364.

Sapolsky R (1992) *Stress, the aging brain and the mechanisms of neuron death*. Cambridge, MA: MIT Press.

Sapolsky RM, Krey LC, & McEwen BS (1986) The neuroendochrinology of stress and aging: The glucocorticoid cascade hypothesis. *Endocrinology Rev*, 7(3):248–301.

Schneider ML, Roughton RC, Koehler AJ, & Lubach GR (1999) Growth and development following prenatal stress exposure in primates: An examination of ontogenetic vulnerability. *Child Dev*, 70(2):263–536.

Schore, AN (1997) Early organization of the nonlinear right brain and development of a predisposition to psychiatric disorders. *Dev Psychopathology*, 9:595–632.

Shin LM, Whalen PJ, Pitman RK, Bush G, Macklin ML, Lasko NB, Orr SP, McInerney SC, & Rauch SL (2001) An fMRI study of anterior cingulate function in posttraumatic stress disorder. *Biol Psychiatry*, 50(12):932–942.

Shulman RG (2001) Functional imaging studies: Linking mind and basic neuroscience. *Am J Psychiatry*, 158:11–20.

Spinelli DN (1987) Plasticity triggering experiences, nature, and the dual genesis of brain structure and function. In N Guzenhauser (Ed.), *Infant stimulation: For whom, what kind, when, and how much?* Skillman, NJ: Johnson & Johnson.

Stein BD, Zima BT, Elliott MN, Burnam MA, Shahinfar A, Fox NA, & Leavitt LA (2001) Violence exposure among school-age children in foster care: relationship to distress symptoms. *J Am Acad Child Adolesc Psychiatry*, 40(5):588–594.

Terr LC (1981) "Forbidden games": Post-traumatic child's play. *J Am Acad Child Adolesc Psychiatry*, 34:547–623.

Terr LC (1991) Childhood traumas: An outline and overview. *Am J Psychiatry*, 148:10–20.

Tooby J & Cosmides L (1990) On the universality of human nature and the uniqueness of the individual: The role of genetics and adaptation. *J Per*, 58:17–68.

Tooby J & Cosmides L (1992) Psychological foundations of culture. In J Barkow, L Cosmides, & J Tooby (Eds.), *The adapted mind* (pp. 19–136). New York: Oxford University Press.

Toth SL, Cicchetti D, Macfie J, & Emde RN (1997) Representations of self and other in the narratives of neglected, physically abused and sexually abused preschoolers. *Dev Psychopathology*, 9:781–796.

Trevarthen C (1978) Secondary intersubjectivity: Confidence, confiding and acts of meaning in the first year. In A Lock (Ed.), *Action, gesture and symbol: The emergence of language* (pp. 183–229). New York: Academic Press.

Tronick EZ & Weinberg MK (1997) Depressed mothers and infants: Failures to form dyadic states of consciousness. In L Murray & P Cooper (Eds.), *Postpartum depression and child development* (pp. 54–81). New York: Guilford Press.

Volkmar F (2001) Diversity and challenges of child psychiatry. *Am J Psychiatry*, 158:987–988.

Vondra J, Barnett D, & Cicchetti D (1989) Perceived and actual competence among maltreated and comparison school children. *Dev Psychopathology*, 1:237–255.

Wang L & Pitts DK (1994) Postnatal development of mesoaccumbens dopamine neurons in the rat: Electrophysiological studies. *Dev Brain Res*, 79:19–28.

Weinstock M (1996) Does prenatal stress impair coping and regulation of hypothalamic–pituitary–adrenal axis? *Neurosci Biobehavioral Rev*, 21(1):1–10.

Weller, EB, Weller RA, & Fristad MA (1995) Bipolar disorder in children: Misdoagnosis, underdiagnosis and future directions. *J Am Acad Child Adolesc Psychiatry*, 34(6):709–715.

Werner, E (1995) Resilience in development. *Curr Dir Psychol Sci*, 4:81–84.

CHAPTER 9

Autism and Pervasive Developmental Disorder

PETER E. TANGUAY

Autistic children were first described by Kanner (1943). Autism was not included in DSM-II (published in 1968), but made its appearance in DSM-III (American Psychiatric Association, 1980) in 1980. Although there have been some changes in the diagnostic features of pervasive developmental disorders in DSM-III-R and DSM-IV, notably the addition to DSM-IV of Asperger's disorder, the diagnostic criteria for autism have remained generally the same. The major features of autism are described in three domains: (1) failure to develop interpersonal relationships and a lack of responsiveness to or interest in people, (2) impairment in communication and imaginative activity, and (3) a markedly restricted repertoire of activities and interests. It is a categorical diagnosis: individuals must show a number of specific criteria, and they must show symptoms from all three domains to receive the diagnosis. In DSM-III it was specified that there should be a *profound* disturbance in social relationships, but in DSM-III-R the term *qualitative impairment* was used to denote severity. In DSM-IV there has been a shift back to requiring that the impairments be severe.

The current diagnostic criteria for autism have a number of important advantages. By requiring that the symptoms must be severe and lead to marked impairment, and must include a minimum number from each domain, the category of autism is likely to include only persons who most clinicians would agree are truly "autistic." This is a nonnegotiable requirement for anyone wishing to study the neurobiology or genetics of autism, or who wishes to do epidemiological research. The DSM-IV field trials established that autism was one of the most robust diagnosis in the nomenclature, with a sensitivity of .82, and a specificity of .87 (Volkmar et al., 1994).

There are persons who have qualitatively similar syndromes to autism, but in whom the symptoms are less severe or fewer in number or not as profoundly disruptive of their lives. Each of the recent DSMs have attempted to provide for this. In DSM-III the diagnosis of *autism–residual state* was reserved for cases where the "full syndrome" was not present; in DSM-III-R and DSM-IV the category of *pervasive developmental disorder not otherwise specified* (PDDNOS) was to be used for persons whose symptoms were not severe or numerous enough to meet the full criteria for *autism*. From a clinical viewpoint this solution has some disadvantages. The criteria for PDDNOS are rather vague, which is quite understandable given the state of our knowledge at the time. Whether we have a better understanding of autism today, as committees assemble to discuss the outlines of "DSM-V," remains to be seen; perhaps it will be DSM-VI before we have enough new knowledge to develop an improved system of diagnosis.

There have been attempts to improve upon the "residual" and "not otherwise specified" categories. The newly defined category of Asperger's disorder, featured in DSM-IV, is one example. The category is reserved for persons who have a profound impairment in interpersonal relationships, but normal language development. My personal experience has been that very few persons with profound social impairment have a history of normal language development prior to 30 months (required in DSM-IV), though many may have normal vocabulary and grammar by age 5 or so. Two categories, *atypical autism* (similar to the residual autism categories in DSM-IV) and *high functioning autism* (e.g., profound social impairments in persons with IQ above 70), have been compared with Asperger's disorder (Eisenmajer et al., 1996; Ghaziuddin et al., 1994; Klin et al., 1995b; Manjiviona & Prior, 1995). Although it is possible to identify statistically significant differences between groups, the clinical significance of the differences is questionable in that they appear to relate mainly to whatever criteria were used to define each of the populations. In most instances the criteria seem to have been subjectively chosen in a somewhat idiosyncratic way.

Wing (1997) proposed a "triad of subtypes" based on social interaction, communication, imagination, and behavior. The subtypes were *aloof* (persons who actively avoid interaction), *passive* (who accept social interaction but do not seek it), and *active but odd* (who accept social interaction but interact in odd and eccentric ways). Volkmar and colleagues (1988) classified autistic persons into Wing's subtypes using questionnaire-based information gathered from teachers or caretakers. Although clinicians were able to reliably group both autistic and nonautistic individuals into the three subtypes, the subtypes were mainly related to IQ. Others have studied Wing's system (Borden & Ollendick, 1994; Castelloe & Dawson, 1993; O'Brien, 1996) and have shown that although it can be reliably used to group persons with pervasive developmental disorder (PDD), the clinical and experimental usefulness of the exercise is uncertain.

Two other categories have been discussed for persons who may have some of the symptoms of autism: nonverbal learning disorder (Rourke, 1989) and multiple complex developmental disorder (Klin et al., 1995a; Towbin et al., 1993). Klin and colleagues (1995b) compared Asperger's disorder with nonverbal learning disorder. They found a robust overlap between the neuropsychological profiles of persons with Asperger's and with nonverbal learning disorder, suggesting that from a clinical viewpoint, the groups were quite similar. Although the clinical features of multiple complex developmental disorder include symptoms of autism, especially the social and interpersonal difficulties, persons with multiple complex developmental disorder also show disturbed anxiety modulation and peculiarities in thinking and language (Klin et al., 1995a; Kumra et al., 1998; Towbin et al., 1993).

For some time it has been recognized that a fundamental problem of classification in autism is that the disorder may not be a *categorical* disorder, but a *spectrum* disorder. There is, in fact, no research data indicating that this is unequivocally so. What may look to us to be a *spectrum* could eventually prove to be the phenotypic manifestations of a concatenation of various genetic abnormalities whose clinical appearance suggests a spectrum. Nonetheless, from a clinical viewpoint, the concept of autism as a spectrum disorder appears interesting. It would allow classification of persons in terms of the degree of their disability, much as one classifies the etiologically heterogeneous group of mentally retarded persons as mild, moderate, severe and profound. Saying that autism is a spectrum disorder, of course, begs the question: a spectrum of what? One possible answer might be: a spectrum of social communication handicaps. But even if this were proven true, an additional conundrum would remain: how would we specify the severity of social communication handicap?

AUTISM AS A DISORDER
OF SOCIAL COMMUNICATION

One of the more important advances in the field of developmental psychology in the past several decades has been to describe the nature of social communication and its development (see Chapter 3). To summarize the earlier material: Children are born with an inborn behavioral propensity to emit facial expressions and to selectively look and listen to the social signals of their immediate caretakers. Within a few months they begin to use a wider variety of social signals as well as being responsive to facial, vocal, gestural, and prosodic cues. This stage of *affective reciprocity* develops into one of *joint attention*, in which they engage in referential communication with their caretakers. By the end of the first year of life children not only have a rich repertoire of nonverbal social communication skills, but they are beginning to show evidence of *theory of mind*, that is, an understanding that other people have minds that are independent from theirs, and from whom they can learn. By age 3 or 4 years children's verbal productions and conversation indicates they are beginning to grasp that people have motives and intentions, and that these can be used to explain and predict their behavior. In contrast, they see objects as significantly different: objects can be acted upon, but do not have motives or intentions. By ages 3–4 years children develop an interest in personal motivation, that is, why do people behave in a particular way, and when do people simulate beliefs as in pretend activities and dissimulation (Baron-Cohen, 1995)? These intuitions represent the beginning of social learning, which will, by adolescence, be represented by the vast store of nonverbal and verbal *social knowledge* crucial to successful social interactions in everyday life. It has been argued that such development implies the interaction of inborn behavioral propensities and social experience, just as language requires a neural and anatomical apparatus capable of learning vocabulary and grammar and producing speech.

A recent study suggests that not all persons show equal skills in recognizing and responding to social signals (Constantino et al., 2000). Using a research instrument, the Social Reciprocity Scale, the authors studied 287 schoolchildren ages 4–14 years. Social reciprocity scores were continuously distributed across subjects. A comparison group of children diagnosed as having autism or Asperger syndrome showed significant impairments in recognition of social cues, interpretation of social cues, and response to social cues.

In keeping with the latter observation, there is increasing evidence that deficits in social communication skills are very important in autism (Baron-Cohen et al., 2001; Shapiro & Hertzig, 1991; Sigman, 1998). The evidence that autistic children do not demonstrate affective reciprocity is largely retrospective. Parents describe the "passivity" of their autistic child as an infant, demonstrated by the child's seldom seeking eye contact, his or her disinterest in playing baby games, and the child's lack of varied facial expression or speech-like babble. Not all children who will later be diagnosed as autistic are said to have been unresponsive; some parents recall their children as being normally responsive until their second year of life. A review of coded home videotapes of 11 autistic and 11 normal children, taken at their first birthday parties, suggests that although late onset of autism may be observed, it may be infrequent (Osterline & Dawson, 1994). Ten of the 11 autistic children were correctly classified on the basis of their lack of pointing, showing objects, looking at others, and orienting to name.

Although children with autism are clearly attached to their mothers and attempt to remain close to them (Dissanayake & Crossley, 1996; Rogers et al., 1991), they fail to engage in the nonverbal social communication interactions typically seen in young children (Baron-Cohen et al., 1993; Sigman & Capps, 1997). They do not spontaneously attempt to engage in joint attention, such as pointing or showing objects (Sigman et al., 1986). They seem not to recognize the emotional and contextual meaning of facial expression, gesture, and nonverbal vocalizations of emotion (Hobson, 1986). Autistic children fail to use the speaker's direction of gaze to orient themselves to objects (Baron-Cohen et al., 1997). In a comparison to children with Down syndrome, autistic persons rarely used emotional gestures, even though they usually could initiate them upon request (Attwood et al., 1988). Persons with autism do not show joint attention (McArthur & Adamson, 1996; Mundy, 1995), and they fail to develop a theory of mind Baron-Cohen, 1995). Deficits in theory of mind have particularly caught the interest of many investigators, who have written extensively on the subject (Baron-Cohen, 1995; Baron-Cohen et al., 1993). Unfortunately, much of the literature has focused on rather narrow aspects of theory of mind (e.g., does the first doll know that the second doll has hidden the desired object in a different place?), rather than on broader issues of pragmatic skills and general social knowledge.

A review of the literature by Bailey and colleagues (1998) concluded that relatives are sometimes affected by difficulties that are conceptually related to autistic behaviors. These ranged in severity from pervasive developmental disorder to abnormalities in only one area of functioning. However, many earlier studies did not use instruments that would be likely to identify social communication behaviors per se. Of those that did, lack of affection, impaired friendships, impaired social play, odd behavior, and impaired conversation were among the characteristic features of impairment. Piven and colleagues (1997), in an example of the latter group, reported finding higher rates of social deficits and stereotypic behaviors in the relatives of families with multiple-incidence autism as compared with families of children with Down syndrome. Piven and his colleagues used a standardized family interview scale that included questions about social communication. Social deficits included lack of spontaneous affection, little to-and-fro social play, limited or no friendships, limited to-and-fro conversation, and frequent inappropriate behavior.

Is autism a spectrum disorder? Although research may someday demonstrate otherwise, at present it seems clinically appropriate to conceptualize it as a unitary disorder whose spectrum of social communication skill deficits are variable.

ASSESSING THE RANGE OF SOCIAL COMMUNICATION DISABILITIES IN AUTISM

How can we operationalize the concept of autism as a spectrum disorder? A recent set of studies (Robertson et al., 1999; Tanguay et al.,

1998) suggest one possible approach, though it leaves many questions unanswered. The investigators chose a cohort of children diagnosed by independent clinicians as having autism, Asperger's disorder, or PDDNOS. The children were evaluated using the Autism Diagnostic Interview (ADI) and the Autism Diagnostic Observation Scale. Data from each of these instruments were subjected to factor analysis. Three factors were identified: *affective reciprocity, joint attention*, and *theory of mind*. The third factor represented disabilities in chatting or in engaging in to-and-fro conversation, a lack of imaginative play, and a lack of social relationships. In the interval since publication of these results, the investigators have raised the number of children with PDD (including autism, Asperger's disorder and PDDNOS) evaluated using the ADI to a total of 115 individuals, and reran the factor analysis. The factor results are shown in Table 9.1. The factor structure was refined to include *nonverbal* and *verbal* joint attention as factors, rather than a single joint attention factor found in the earlier work. A description of how this method can be applied to specific children has been published (Tanguay et al., 2001). More recently, Tadevosyan-Layfer and colleagues (2003) reported a principal components analysis of the Autism Diagnostic Interview—Revised (ADI-R) for 292 persons with autism. Because of their larger cohort they were able to include many more variables in their study than had been included in the previously referenced work. They found that six variable clusters emerged: spoken language, compulsions, developmental milestones, savant skills, sensory aversions, and social intent. Social intent appears to be similar to the familiar social communication domain, whereas the other domains may represent important, but somewhat independent features of the symptoms found in autism.

SYMPTOMS ARE NOT PATHOGNOMONIC OF A SPECIFIC DIAGNOSIS

Watkins and colleagues (1988) studied symptom development in 17 children who met the DSM-III criteria for schizophrenia with onset before 10 years of age. Detailed psychiatric histories and records of previous mental status examinations were available for many of the children. Using a follow-back design, symptom development was

TABLE 9.1. Social Communication Domains and their Associated ADI Variables

Affective reciprocity
- Offers comfort to others in distress
- Greets others with pleasure
- Offers to share toys/food with others
- Normal range of facial expressions
- Shares others' excitement
- Seeks to share enjoyment with others

Emotional joint attention
- Responsive social smile
- Seeks eye contact with others
- Affectionate to others
- Directs others' attention to toys/objects in which he or she has an interest

Verbal joint attention
- Engages in social chat
- Carries on a reciprocal conversation

Social imagination/play
- Uses social gestures
- Imitative play—social games
- Interest in other children
- Responsive to other children's approach
- Imaginative play alone; creative use of actions and objects
- Imaginative play with peers
- Group play with peers

Note. The variables were grouped into the four domains using a factor analysis of data from 115 cases independently diagnosed as meeting the DSM-IV criteria for PDD by two expert clinicians.

rated at four ages using a DSM-III Symptom Rating Scale and the Achenbach Child Behavior Checklist. Results revealed a gradual developmental unfolding of a broad spectrum of symptoms affecting social, cognitive, sensory, and motor functioning that had begun many years before the appearance of schizophrenic symptoms. Symptoms of autism prior to age 6 were found in 39% of the sample. Initially, the children in question appeared to be developing normally, but after 4 years of age their development was grossly disrupted and they began to be "autistic." Previous epidemiological, family, and twin studies have shown that schizophrenia and autism appear to be unrelated genetically (Rutter & Schopler,

1987), leading to a conclusion that developmental issues may account for the findings of Watson and colleagues. If one develops a brain disorder such as schizophrenia early in life, the symptoms are likely to reflect disruptions in developmental tasks that are developmentally tied to that age. In the case of children 3–6 years of age, these tasks encompass learning the social skills and gaining the intuitive knowledge necessary for everyday social interaction. In the case of children with autism, the symptoms represent a failure in development, but in the case of the children with early-onset schizophrenia, the symptoms may be manifestation of a failure or a regression in developmental progress. In a parallel fashion, children who have undergone extreme social isolation and deprivation (Rutter et al., 1999) may also show signs of autism, though these tend to abate once the children are placed in therapeutic foster homes. It has also been reported that a lack of "theory of mind" and signs of poor pragmatic skills can be found in persons with Down syndrome (Yirmiya et al., 1996, 1998; Zelazo et al., 1996) and adult-onset schizophrenia (Mazza et al., 2001; Pickup & Frith, 2001).

CONCLUSION

Children typically develop motor, language, social, and intellectual skills along a pathway that is driven by inborn propensities and by experience. Children with mental retardation and autism fail to reach expected developmental milestones. A failure of language, social, and intellectual development is likely to result in the DSM-IV symptoms of classical autism. If intellectual and language skills unfold normally but social skills fail to be learned, the child may be diagnosed as having high-functioning autism or Asperger's disorder. For any one person, it is not the symptoms per se that are of importance, but the meaning of the symptoms in terms of whether they represent an arrest of development or a regression in development. The history of the present illness may need to be augmented with relevant family history ("Is there anyone else in the family—grandparent, aunt, uncle, cousin—who has had a similar disorder?") in order to begin to reach a correct diagnosis and an understanding of the nature of a particular child's problems.

REFERENCES

American Psychiatric Association (1980) *Diagnostic and statistical manual of mental disorders* (3rd ed.). Washington, DC: Author.

Attwood A, Frith U, & Hermelin B (1988) The understanding and use of interpersonal gestures by autistic and Down's syndrome children. *J Autism Dev Disord*, 18:241–257.

Bailey A, Palferman S, Heavey L, & Le Couteur A (1998) Autism: The phenotype in relatives. *J Autism Devl Disord*, 28:369–392.

Baron-Cohen S (1995) *Mindblindness*. Cambridge, MA: MIT Press.

Baron-Cohen S, Baldwin DA, & Crowson M (1997) Do children with autism use the speaker's direction of gaze strategy to crack the code of language? *Child Dev*, 68:48–57.

Baron-Cohen S, Tager-Flusberg H, & Cohen D (1993) *Understanding other minds*. New York: Oxford University Press.

Baron-Cohen S, Wheelwright S, Skinner R, Martin J, & Clubley E (2001) The autism-spectrum quotient (AQ): Evidence from Asperger syndrome/high-functioning autism, males and females, scientists and mathematicians. *J Autism Dev Disord*, 31:5–17.

Borden MC & Ollendick TH (1994) An examination of the validity of social subtypes in autism. *J Autism Dev Disord*, 24:23–37.

Castelloe P & Dawson G (1993) Subclassification of children with autism and pervasive developmental disorder: A questionnaire based on Wing's subgrouping scheme. *J Autism Dev Disord*, 23:229–241.

Constantino JN, Przybeck T, Friesen D, & Todd RD (2000) Reciprocal social behavior in children with and without pervasive developmental disorders. *J Dev Behav Pediatr*, 21:2–11.

Dissanayake C & Crossley SA (1996) Proximity and sociable behaviours in autism: Evidence for attachment. *J Child Psychol Psychiatry*, 37:149–156.

Eisenmajer R, Prior M, Leekam S, Wing L, Gould J, Welham M, & Ong B (1996) Comparison of clinical symptoms in autism and Asperger's disorder. *J Am Acad Child Adolesc Psychiatry*, 35:523–531.

Ghaziuddin M, Butler E, Tsai L, & Ghaziuddin N (1994) Is clumsiness a marker for Asperger syndrome? *J Intell Disab Res*, 38:519–527.

Hobson P (1986) The autistic child's appraisal of emotion. *J Child Psychol Psychiatry*, 27:21–342.

Kanner L (1943) Autistic disturbances of affective contact. *Nerv Child*, 2:17–250.

Klin A, Mayes LC, Volkmar FR, & Cohen DJ (1995a) Multiplex developmental disorder. *J Dev Behav Pediatr*, 16:7–11.

Klin A, Volkmar FR, Sparrow SS, Cicchetti DV, & Rourke BP (1995b) Validity and neuropsychological characterization of Asperger syndrome: Convergence with nonverbal learning disabilities syndrome. *J Child Psychol Psychiatry*, 36:1127–1140.

Kumra S, Jacobsen LK, Lenane M, Zahn TP, Wiggs E, Alaghband-Rad J, Castellanos FX, Frazier JA, McKenna K, Gordon CT, Smith A, Hamburger S, & Rapoport JL (1998) "Multidimensionally impaired disorder": is it a variant of very early-onset schizophrenia? *J Am Acad Child Adolesc Psychiatry,* 37:91–99.

Manjiviona J & Prior M (1995) Comparison of Asperger syndrome and high-functioning autistic children on a test of motor impairment. *J Autism Dev Disord,* 25:23–39.

Mazza M, De Risio A, Surian L, Roncone R, & Casacchia M (2001) Selective impairments of theory of mind in people with schizophrenia. *Schizophr Res,* 47:299–308.

McArthur D & Adamson LB (1996) Joint attention in preverbal children: Autism and developmental language disorder. *J Autism Dev Disord,* 26:481–496.

Mundy P (1995) Joint attention and social-emotional approach behavior in children with autism. *Dev Psychopathology,* 7:63–82.

O'Brien, SK (1996) The validity and reliability of the Wing Subgroups Questionnaire. *J Autism Dev Disord,* 26:321–335.

Osterline J & Dawson G (1994) Early recognition of children with autism: A study of first birthday home videotapes. *J Autism Dev Disord,* 24:247–257.

Pickup GJ & Frith CD (2001) Theory of mind impairments in schizophrenia: Symptomatology, severity and specificity. *Psychological Med,* 31:207–220.

Piven J, Palmer P, Jacobi D, Childress D, & Arndt S (1997) Broader autism phenotype: Evidence from a family history study of multiple-incidence autism families. *Am J Psychiatry,* 154:185–190.

Robertson J, Tanguay P, L'Ecuyer S, Sims A, & Waltrip C (1999) Domains of social communication handicap in autism spectrum disorder. *J Am Acad Child Adolesc Psychiatry,* 38:738–745.

Rogers SJ, Ozonoff S, & Maslin CC (1991) A comparative study of attachment behavior in young children with autism or other psychiatric disorders. *J Am Acad Child Adolesc Psychiatry,* 30:483–488.

Rourke BP (1989) *Non-verbal learning disabilities: The syndrome and the model.* New York: Guilford Press.

Rutter M, Andersen-Wood L, Beckett C, Bredenkamp D, Castle J, Groothues C, Kreppner J, Keaveney L, Lord C, & O'Connor TG (1999) Quasi-autistic patterns following severe early global privation: English and Romanian Adoptees (ERA) study team. *J Child Psychol Psychiatry Allied Disciplines,* 40:537–549.

Rutter M & Schopler E (1987) Autism and pervasive developmental disorders: Concepts and diagnostic issues. *J Autism Dev Disord,* 17:159–186.

Shapiro T & Hertzig ME (1991) Social deviance in autism: A central integrative failure as a model for social nonengagement. *Psychiatr Clin North Am,* 14:19–32.

Sigman M (1998) The Emanuel Miller Memorial Lecture 1997. Change and continuity in the development of children with autism. *J Child Psychol Psychiatry Allied Disciplines,* 39:817–827.

Sigman M & Capps L (1997) *Children with autism: A developmental perspective.* Cambridge, MA: Harvard University Press.

Sigman M, Mundy P, Sherman T, & Ungerer J (1986) Social interactions of autistic, mentally retarded and normal children and their caregivers. *J Child Psychol Psychiatry,* 27:647–656.

Tadevosyan-Layfer O, Dowd M, Mankoski R, Winklosky B, Putnam S, McGrath L, Tager-Flusberg H, & Folstein S (2003) A principal components analysis of the Autism Diagnostic Interview—Revised. *J Am Acad Child Adolesc Psychiatry,* 42:864–872.

Tanguay PE, Robertson J, & Derrick A (1998) A dimensional classification of autism spectrum disorder by social communication domains. *J Am Acad Child Adolesc Psychiatry,* 37:271–277.

Tanguay PE, Robertson J, & Derrick A (2001) A system of classification for autism spectrum disorder. *J Dev Learning Disord,* 5:95–106.

Towbin KE, Dykens EM, Pearson GS, & Cohen DJ (1993) Conceptualizing "borderline syndrome of childhood" and "childhood schizophrenia" as a developmental disorder. *J Am Acad Child Adolesc Psychiatry,* 32:775–782.

Volkmar FR, Cohen DJ, Bregman JD, Hooks MY, & Stevenson JM (1988) An examination of social typologies in autism. *J Am Acad Child Adolesc Psychiatry,* 28:82–86.

Volkmar FR, Klin A, Siegel B, Szatmari P, Lord C, Campbell M, Freeman BJ, Cicchetti DV, Rutter M, & Kline W (1994) Field trial for autistic disorder in DSM-IV. *Am J Psychiatry,* 151:1361–1367.

Watson J, Asarnow R, & Tanguay P (1988) Symptom development in childhood onset schizophrenia. *J Child Psychol Psychiatry,* 29:865–878.

Wing L (1997) The autistic spectrum *Lancet,* 350:1761–1766.

Yirmiya N, Erel O, Shaked M, & Solomonica-Levi D (1998) Meta-analyses comparing theory of mind abilities of individuals with autism, individuals with mental retardation, and normally developing individuals. *Psychological Bull,* 124:283–307.

Yirmiya N, Solomonica-Levi D, Shulman C, & Pilowsky T (1996) Theory of mind abilities in individuals with autism, Down syndrome, and mental retardation of unknown etiology: The role of age and intelligence. *J Child Psychol Psychiatry Allied Disciplines,* 37:1003–1014.

Zelazo PD, Burack JA, Benedetto E, & Frye D (1996) Theory of mind and rule use in individuals with Down's syndrome: A test of the uniqueness and specificity claims. *J Child Psychol Psychiatry,* 37:479–484.

CHAPTER 10

Recommendations for DSM-V

PENNY KNAPP *and* PETER S. JENSEN

The architects of the DSM-III, -III-R and -IV took pains to avoid the pitfalls of speculation, abstraction, and projection by seeking clinical consensus on the phenomenology of mental disorders. Yet avoiding one set of pitfalls has led to others: the DSM has been used to reify phenomena that may be diverse, to arbitrate who may and who may not receive treatment, and to constrain research inquiry to the specific terms of the written descriptive categories. As a manual of observable mental disorders, it describes these disorders as they have reached their full manifestations. In the interests of clarity and scientific credibility, the predispositions, primordia, and prodromes of the disorders are not described. Developmental factors are minimized, so the manifestations of emotions and behaviors of children whose development is at risk for deviance are far less likely to be included. Relationships, crucial for social survival and evolutionary adaptation of a social animal, are not described, even though behaviors, such as aggression and paranoia, with powerful impacts on relationships, are listed as symptoms. For young children, whose self-organization springs from family relationships, whose personal experience suffused with those relationships has not been built upon with later life experiences, this omission invites descriptions of symptoms that are diagnostically mysterious.

Much more difficult than the project of criticizing our current

162

diagnostic system is the project of creating a better one. What should a diagnostic system be able to do for us? It should be descriptive, of course, but it should also be predictive, and it should guide treatment, whether treatment be narrowly construed as the suppression of disturbing symptoms or widely construed as freeing the patient to achieve his or her developmental optimum. It should assist the diagnostician to discriminate between disorder definitions as social constructions or as diseases of the mind, either of which could be subject to evolution or adaptation. It should provide guidelines for deciding which persons who are either suffering or causing suffering will qualify as "cases" for treatment. These guidelines should help the treating professional to understand whether treatment is for symptoms that create specific functional impairment (endangering adaptability), or global functional impairment (requiring support from family or society), or both—thus assisting the society to adapt better to meet the needs of all its members. Ideally it will open the doors, as the DSM has sought to do, to improved scientific description of phenomenology and will catalyze research efforts in the field. To accomplish this, particularly in the understanding of mental disorders in children, there is no alternative to going beyond the current phenotypes, and the subtypes of those phenotypes, to include two dimensions essential to human adaptive capacity: development and relationships.

An individual's symptomatology may betray adaptive strain, developmental skew, and/or toxic relationships. A recent phenomenon in diagnosis using the DSM system is the proliferation of diagnoses of comorbid conditions. Reliance on the concept of *comorbidity* betrays the strain of using the DSM to describe emotional and behavioral phenomena, especially in children. This practical skew in the application of the DSM as a tool is an indication that it fails to explain emerging brain activities in their context. Proliferation of the use of comorbid diagnoses is a faltering effort to repair the troubled relationship between the DSM system and the research, reimbursement, and social policy communities.

DIAGNOSTIC COMORBIDITY: A ROUND CONCEPT IN A SQUARE BOX

Comorbidity, like temperament, is readily observable, but current descriptions fail to explain it. It has been reified as a metadiagnostic construct that seeks to fill descriptive gaps, to improve the precision of treatment, and to entitle patients to care even if they cannot be fitted onto the procrustean bed of the current DSM system. Just as changing needs for survival and adaptation over time will mold the brain in different ways through natural selection, the different symptom clusters that form our diagnostic system today have emerged as to-and-fro derivatives of this process. As we seek to apply a neo-Darwinian or adaptive model to the clinical problems we face every day, comorbidity, a symptomatic complication of the diagnostic system, or an unwanted "side effect" of the system, may point us in a useful direction. The construct of comorbidity may be a reflection of this exquisite sensitivity in the complex interactions of inherent and adaptive systems that regulate cognitive and emotional states.

Comorbidity, the simultaneous occurrence of two or more unrelated conditions (Caron & Rutter, 1991), was a surprising and unwanted finding in early epidemiological surveys. The fact that *clinical* samples are comorbid was taken for granted. But studies of broader community populations were expected to parse this phenomenon by providing relatively pure diagnostic samples. Instead, although comorbidity was found less frequently in epidemiological than in clinical samples, its existence in community samples exceeded what one could expect from chance. It is this finding that has moved us from the search for the "single diagnosis" to a consideration of the meaning of the complicated interaction among diagnoses (Lewinsohn et al., 1995). Even more unsettling, comorbidity often involves both internalizing and externalizing problems, challenging the generally held belief that diagnoses could be sorted into relatively independent and separate clusters (McConaughy & Achenbach, 1994).

When two or more diagnoses coexist in the same child, there are several possible explanations: (1) they represent conditions that are separate and distinct from each other; (2) they represent the *same* condition, behind the camouflage that makes them *appear* to be different; (3) they represent different developmental stages of the same condition occurring simultaneously; or (4) they are separate symptom manifestations of a common underlying condition. Because the first possibility, that comorbid conditions are separate and distinct from each other, is now untenable for many of our comorbidity findings, and the second possibility either an error in diagnosis or a boundary artifact, let us consider the third and fourth possibilities, the vertical and horizontal manifestations of comorbidity, now called successive comorbidity and concurrent comorbidity (Angold et al., 1999a).

First, we consider successive comorbidity. It is known that child and adolescent psychopathology changes with age. Oppositional defiant disorder (ODD) becomes conduct disorder (CD) becomes antisocial personality disorder (ASP)—a pathway that narrows over time, possibly reflecting developmental sequences of a single underlying pathological process. Each diagnosis may represent a vulnerability factor for the next successive stage (i.e., ODD typically precedes CD, and CD typically precedes ASP in adulthood). But the sequence is more complicated when attention-deficit/hyperactivity disorder (ADHD) enters the picture. Although ADHD may appear to serve as a stage in the development of CD (and later ASP), some have suggested another more serious scenario: only youngsters with *comorbid* ADHD and ODD develop the most severe or persistent form of CD, with earlier onset and higher levels of aggression. The exact nature of the interlocking connections between these conditions has yet to be mapped from longitudinal studies (Faraone et al., 1997). The phenomenon of comorbidity, then, may reflect an underlying global psychopathological factor that assumes a more specific symptomatic form with increasing differentiation at successive stages of development in vulnerable children.

The phenomenon of comorbidity may reflect a lost developmental concept, the evolving stages of disorder compressed in time so that they appear concurrent. In diagnosing comorbidity, we may be seeing the end of one pathological stage and the beginning of another. After all, successive stages of disease are recognized in general medicine. First ankle edema, then dyspnea, then cyanosis, all reflecting symptomatic stages of a single disease, congestive heart failure, formerly termed "dropsy." Yet the underlying pathophysiology uniting them remained hidden for centuries. As long as we cannot see underlying pathophysiological connections, we will continue to diagnose edema or cyanosis instead of congestive heart failure, mistaking symptoms for disease.

Just as successive, or the vertical expression of, comorbidity may suggest certain developmental interlocking connections, the term "concurrent comorbidity" assumes a horizontal spectrum of related overlapping conditions, phenotypic variability from a single underlying genotype, if you will. And as we move toward a better understanding of genetic susceptibility in humans, we may relate the comorbidity of Tourette syndrome and obsessive–compulsive disorder to an overlapping spectrum of symptoms, expressing phenotypic variability of an underlying genotype.

Evolution has taught us that adaptation does not require millennia or even centuries. It can occur concurrently with life experience as a result of cultural pressures. Dark-winged moths won out over light-winged ones in the industrial areas of England because their dark color protected them from predator birds when they lighted on soot-darkened tree trunks. But in rural England, where there was no black soot on the bark of trees, the opposite survival pattern was seen (Kettlewell, 1956). If one assumes a generalized underlying pathophysiology (e.g., undifferentiated anxiety/depression), it cannot only be viewed as potential for *successive* comorbidity in the same individual, but can also be seen as different expression in individuals depending on cultural context favoring one set of symptoms or the other (e.g., the dark-winged or light-winged moth), or concurrent comorbidity.

Comorbidity has forced us to redefine the natural boundaries between diagnoses. Truly separate disorders should rarely overlap. Significant overlap probably suggests successive developmental stage-related or concurrent spectrum-related conditions. We must go beyond simply generating more symptom lists and diagnoses and stop to examine these interrelationships. Using new conceptual models, for example, the neo-Darwinian, the interaction between clinical, epidemiological, and molecular reasoning can expose these hidden connections. Comorbidity, originally seen as a nuisance contaminating our modern diagnostic system, may offer a key to solving the puzzle of the relationship between surface symptoms and the underlying pathophysiology. It may create new diagnostic continuities from what have appeared to be chance associations. When we have understood these new continuities, we will then be challenged to explain the remaining discontinuities. True understanding will be signaled by newer, but fewer, diagnostic categories, not developing more and more subtypes of those we now employ.

RECOMMENDATIONS FOR DSM-V
AND FUTURE RESEARCH

To address the assessment challenges noted in previous chapters, we close with a series of recommendations, starting first with general recommendations that are applicable across the various purposes of classification and mental disorder determination, followed by recommendations specific to mental disorder determination for "pragmatic" reasons (e.g., unmet need), and ending with recommendations for mental disorder determination for scientific purposes of syndrome identification, etiologic studies, risk factor determination, treatment trials, the expected clinical courses, and outcome studies.

Disorder Definitions as Social Constructions

The DSM is a categorical model, written to guide the clinician to pick, among diagnostic categories, the diagnosis(es) that best fit the patient. However, as Eisenberg (1995) has noted, researchers and clinicians must be cautioned to avoid "reifying" the disorder definitions. Definitions of disorders should not be construed as "things as they truly are," but as simplifications and boundaries around which we demarcate and simplify various aspects of nature for certain purposes, in this case, to study or treat them and communicate our understanding to others. We must understand that the problems that characterize the definition of psychiatric disorders also characterize many other aspects of medicine, such as the definitions of juvenile-onset diabetes, fibromyalgia, or hypertension, all of which rely on the expression of a minimum set of signs or symptoms, of sufficient severity, over a period time of sufficient length, in order to make the diagnosis. None of the definitions is final, but each constitutes a hypothesis based on the available knowledge at a paricular point in time. As research yields new findings and understanding, changes in classification should be expected, just as the definitions of HIV have rapidly changed over the last two decades as a function of new research. The routes to understanding and the implications of such understanding need not be uniform, inasmuch as disease processes and outcomes are highly variable. Some of the DSM disorders are best understood as specific syndromes, others might be better characterized as final common pathways.

"Caseness" for What?

One virtue of the DSM system is that it allows consensus about the definition of disorders, so that investigators of third-party payors may recognize whether a person with particular symptoms is or is not a "case" for inclusion in a study or for billing for services.

"Caseness" is a tactical necessity for research or for service. To avoid confusing the means and ends of various classification systems, when one offers suggestions or improvements for definitions of mental disorder, the first question asked by informed clinicians and investigators should be, "Caseness for what?" Such a strategy may help avoid unnecessary debates, such as confusing the means of determining a best fit cutoff score with the goal of identifying underlying disease processes, or the means of finding a biologic marker with the goal of determining who really needs care. For our current DSM, this may lead to dramatic reconsideration of how we have combined these two purposes in the more recent versions of the DSMs. As an alternative, we may wish to consider dividing and simplifying the current tasks of DSM, so that one form of classification system is used to determine who needs care (that is, whose condition is severe enough to warrant the expenditure of public resources) or to identify the kind of treatment needed, versus another classification system designed to enable the necessary research descriptions of the phenomenology of mental disorders. Because we consider these two aims fundamentally different, we offer additional recommendations for determining caseness, separating our subsequent recommendations according to their different purposes.

Mental Disorder Determination for Medical Necessity and Need for Treatment

Underlying the decision about whether treatment is needed is the question of prognosis. Ideally, diagnosis offers a prediction about prognosis, and treatment can improve the odds of a better prognosis. However, in childhood, especially in early childhood, change is rapid and predicting the continuity of a disorder over time is difficult (Emde & Robinson, 2002; Lavigne et al., 1998). Simple lines of causation, especially with regard to biologically based brain functions, are less clear in childhood, as multiple etiological factors operate in the experience-dependent construction of brain regulation, each involving interactions of biology and environment, through the child's experience. We suggest that in order to know whether a case or its attendant impairment is *clinically significant*, the need to get into the mind of the clinician is inescapable. What does "clinically significant" mean? A condition of the typical severity that normally comes to the attention of clinicians? If so, which clinicians? How would such definitions vary as a function of the particular culture, time, and available resources? We suggest that such a definition will and must remain quite fluid, based on just these factors.

It should be noted that definitions of mental disorder, as outlined earlier, are relatively culture specific. Within a given society, the impact of cultural factors on diagnosis may operate in variable ways. This is because cultures vary in the tasks required and the demands placed on individuals. This, in turn, is likely to impact clinicians' judgments of impairment and whether a given condition should be accorded mental disorder status. For example, Alarcon (1995) has noted that less favorable diagnoses are frequently applied to individuals in poor ethnic communities, and any diagnostic system (including DSM-IV) runs the risk of becoming a vehicle of an ethnocentric view of mental disorder. Current efforts to infuse cultural competence into mental health systems encounter an obstacle in the DSM, which lists behaviors as symptoms without regard to their societal or cultural appropriateness for the individual. Informative cross-cultural studies are recommended, so that one could examine groups of clinicians and cases from various cultures and conduct some sort of "discrepancy interview" to determine why a particular person would be deemed a case in one culture but not another. For example, in a society with a less advanced schooling system and few academic demands on children, children with milder forms of ADHD might not merit mental disorder status in that particular society, as they may be better able to get by than if they were in an intensely competitive school system where more demands were imposed upon attention, concentration, and follow-through. To avoid such difficulties, even within a given society that has merged a variety of different cultures, there may be a need for publication of a casebook that presents examples or characteristics of how a given condition is manifested in different cultural subgroups.

Mental Disorder Determination for Scientific Description of Phenomenology

Future studies, whose goal is precise scientific description, must adopt a higher standard than was acceptable in the past. Just as with clinical studies whereby one seeks to determine efficacious therapies, epidemiological studies whose goal is to identify the causes, correlates, and courses of specific disorders must develop procedures that more closely approximate a longitudinal expert all data (LEAD) standard (Torrens et al., 2004). This does not necessarily mean that clinicians must be utilized for epidemiologic studies, but their input and examination of the validity of cases of specific disorders should not rely alone on the blind application of DSM criteria, regardless of informant (Bird et al., 2000). Thus, procedures must be developed to resolve discrepancies in the diagnostic information derived from multiple informants, with a systematic attempt to arrive at a more valid synthesis of discrepant reports. Some preliminary efforts in this regard have been reported (Jensen et al., 1999b), but such methods are in their infancy. Other strategies, which rely on "discrepancy interviews" or that make modifications to diagnostic procedures to reduce the likelihood of informants' misunderstanding the questions, have been developed (Edelbrock et al., 1999; Jensen & Edelbrock, 1999), but these have not been tested across multiple centers nor have they enjoyed broad use. More sustained efforts in this regard are needed.

Other approaches to these issues might usefully employ conceptual analysis. Given the goals of scientific description of phenomena, the relatively arbitrary thresholds for symptoms as outlined in the DSM should not restrict investigators from careful assessment of measurement of what might otherwise be "subthreshold" conditions. Not only does this strategy appear to make good sense in areas such as adult depressive disorders (Kendler & Gardner, 1998), but even disorders such as autism may have more dimensional components that are expressed in family members who would not at all be considered for the diagnosis of autism, nor even subthreshold states (Piven & Palmer, 1999). Because the underlying processes that eventually culminate in disorder are often not fully expressed, failure to capture the entire range of psychological and behavioral phenomena in a given person's presenting picture, even when these phenomena are considered "normal," may result in a lack of precision, as well as stultification of scientific progress.

Among DSM-IV disorders applied to children and adolescents, some are driven predominantly by biological factors (e.g., autism), others, although they have associated biological diatheses, arise principally from experience (e.g., posttraumatic stress disorder), and many (e.g., mood disorders, ADHD) are heterogeneous; individuals with these diagnoses differ as to what part is contributed by an underlying diathesis and what part has resulted from life experience.

Better descriptions of the person's familial and social environments are essential (e.g., Baker et al., 2003) in order to pursue the goal of more precise scientific description of the underlying phenomena, as this requires considering all the critical variables. For the DSM-V this will take into account the likelihood that most disorders arise as a function of a particular biological substrate that unfolds in the context of certain current and historical factors within the environment. Thus, Sadler and Hulgus (1994) note that because the current DSM systems do not always fully account for and specify the relevance of interactional data, they fit the needs of a biological psychiatry much better than family-interactional, sociological, developmental, or life history models of disorder, a point also acknowledged by Frances and colleagues (1994). Just as neglect of the dimensions of behavioral and emotional phenomena will hinder progress, failure to fully describe contextual phenomena will likely preclude important discoveries of the disease processes underlying most DSM disorders, even after genetic factors have been more fully specified.

For example, in a study of children in Appalachia, Angold and colleagues (1999b) found that a substantial proportion of children were "impaired yet undiagnosed"; that is, they evidenced substantial impairment yet did not meet criteria for any DSM-defined disorder. Interestingly, most of these cases met criteria for "V code" conditions, especially those involving interactional disturbances in the home. These interactional influences may be especially important for children, given the evidence that it is precisely these types of transactional processes that related to persistence of disorder (Ferdinand & Verhulst, 1995; Lavigne et al., 1998). Capturing an adequate description of such phenomena will be necessary if we are to understand the disease processes and learn how particular disorders evolve and consolidate over time.

Diagnosis in the Service of Adaptation: Treatment Considerations

Diagnosis without a hope of treatment may satisfy us intellectually, but it should unsettle us from a moral or practical perspective. Treatment, for developing persons, must influence their development favorably (Connors et al., 2001; Wells et al., 2000). All patients should be regarded as being in the midst of development, but the development of children and adolescents is rapid and often fateful, and it happens perforce in the context of their intimate relationships. For a diagnostic system to describe the symptoms of children in a way that permits their treatment to be effective, it must incorporate developmental and relationship factors. Moreover, only diagnostic systems with a developmental foundation that acknowledges the concepts of temperament and social communication, and characterizes reciprocal behaviors with significant others, can measure change in children. This is necessary for us to decide if treatment has been effective in changing the young person's developmental trajectory.

For example, understanding the similarity of activation of circuitry between separation anxiety and panic disorder, distinct from that activated by fear or social phobia, guides us to more effective pharmacological approaches, as described in Chapter 4. It also points toward possible early interventions that influence the plasticity of systems mediating these conditions. A diagnostic system that included understanding of the evolutionary and developmental aspects of different anxiety disorders would inform and justify both pharmacological and nonpharmacological interventions and provide a measure of their effect on the regulation of anxiety earlier in the child's development.

Breaking Apart the Phenotype

Given the underlying problems of categorical versus dimensional assessments of psychopathology, as well as the lack of evidence that the DSMs have truly "carved nature at the joints," we suggest that more careful descriptions and fine-grained distinctions of the various components of current diagnoses are necessary. This process of careful dissection and description of the behavioral and emotional phenomena has been described as "breaking apart the phenotype," that is, searching for the more critical components of behavioral and emotional functioning that presumably more closely map onto underlying disease processes. A good case in point is the category of learning disability, for which the previous decade of research demonstrated that traditional definitions did not identify any stable underlying deficit. Learning disabilities are now seen as dimensional, not categorical, conditions, as research has not identified specific markers that qualitatively distinguish different types of disability in learning from other patterns of "underachievement" (Fletcher et al., 2003; Shaywitz et al., 1992). Concomitantly, recent advances have identified a critical component manifested in cases of dyslexia, characterized by difficulties in phonologic awareness.

Shaywitz and Shaywitz (2003) have also analyzed converging evidence from functional magnetic resonance imaging, positron emission tomography, and magnetoencephalography pointing to differences between dyslexic readers and readers without impairment in the temporo–parieto–occipetal brain regions, and failure in dyslexic readers, of proper function during reading in the left hemisphere posterior brain system. Gender differences in functional organization of the brain for language are also confirmed. Several teams of investigators have now replicated findings linking deficits in phonological awareness to chromosome 6 (Fisher et al., 2002; Gayan et al., 1999; Gringorenko et al., 2003). The same distinction has proven useful in developing new approaches to treatment, based on models of neuroplasticity and developmental neurobiology (Knopick et al., 2002; Tallal et al., 1996). Other cases in point are easily found among various medical disorders, such as the example involving thalassemia noted in Chapter 2 (page 20). In such instances, knowledge of the underlying disease process (point mutations in the hemoglobin molecule) may allow intensification of specificity about what constitutes "cases" of disorder, as well as more effective prevention or earlier intervention. Although this is an as yet unattained hope in the instance of mental disorders, the possibility that some forms of schizophrenia may reflect disturbances in neuronal migration during early periods of brain development (Arnold, 1999; Kendler et al., 1987) or that some instances of autism reflect failure of normal pruning processes during the first years of life (Courchesne, 2002; Howard et al., 2000) may yet be realized in the next few years as the rapid advances in the understanding of precise molecular mechanisms progress.

The possibility for substantive advances need not await neuroscientific findings alone. Some investigators have suggested that the strategy of examining various subgroups (e.g., age of onset, the possibility of gender-associated symptoms, neuropsychological test findings) may offer the possibility of similar gains. For example, for ADHD, Jensen and colleagues (Jensen, 2001; Jensen et al., 2001) have recommended that future studies of ADHD carefully tease out various subgroups as a function of differences on neuropsychological tests. Similarly, promising strategies have been noted with other forms of subdivision and classification—for example, history of perinatal trauma (Biederman et al., 1996; Rosa Neto et al., 2002) or comorbidity (Jensen et al., 1999a)—or other methods, such as neuroimaging (Kates et al., 2002; Keefe, 1995), as well as other disorders (Leckman et al., 2001). Of course, one potential obstacle to this objective is the possibility that children's central nervous systems are not yet finalized enough to allow such specific subtypes to be identified, as additional processes that yet determine the final form of specific disorders have not yet occurred.

Thus, the "lumpers" and "splitters" among us must scrutinize each other's assumptions and find means to bring various components of critical thought to bear on current diagnostic and nosologic practices. Among current diagnostic categories, we must carefully examine subgroups à la the methods of Robins and Guze (1970) and further refine our categories as evidence proceeds. Similarly, when faced with lack of evidence for separate diagnostic categories, reconsideration of their presumed discrimination may be required. Moreover, even when cases appear similar in terms of current behavioral phenomena, we must remember that it is likely that "cases" become cases through quite different routes. Two phenotypically similar persons may actually represent two different populations—one that is drawn from the high end of normal processes, another that reflects some disease process—just as some tall persons appear to reflect a disorder in growth hormone production and others do not reflect any identifiable disease process. Characteristics that may identify etiologically meaningful subgroups might actually lie in the past history of the person, rather than in any current phenotypic expression—for example, early- versus late-onset conduct disorder.

One possible strategy to help eliminate the "noise" in the search for disease processes might be to eliminate cases from studies in which there are clear differences in onset, course, or likely etiology. As a simple example, if one is attempting to study ADHD illness processes, including ADHD cases with onset only after head trauma and no family history may lead to some confusion in findings. Although some discoveries may be made through examining the similarities and differences between such subgroups, lumping such different "types" as a general rule may obscure any meaningful findings in many studies, such as an investigation of risk factors, comparing depression and ADHD. As another example, studies of biological factors as *primary* etiological processes for conduct disorder in a sample of youth living in an environment ridden with psychosocial stressors linked to substantial risk for conduct disorder, may be ill advised, unless perhaps one is attempting to examine environmental effects on biological outcomes in those who develop persistent conduct disorder. This is not an issue of "political correctness"; rather, the problem turns simply on the signal-to-noise ratio and the ability to design an efficient experiment with likely pay off. Including cases of likely differing etiologies in a study of disease processes could obscure findings, unless the study design is meant to specifically address the etiologic questions by comparing the specific subgroups. Yet another example: If there are good conceptual reasons to separate out "predatory" versus "reactive" aggression, lumping may be unwise until a substantial body of evidence has accumulated that shows that the distinction is meaningless—that is, that it conveys no meaningful additional information (etiology, treatment, prognosis) beyond the commonsense meaning of the two adjectives.

Unfortunately, all too often it is unclear as to what the etiological factors are or might be. With children, however, there may exist opportunities for subgrouping that are not as readily achieved when studying adults. Given the child's rapid rate of growth and development, these developmental processes may be considered as a potential discriminator of differing processes, such as with early- and late-onset conduct disorder. Here, differing trajectories of disorder and symptomatology may belie qualitatively different underlying disease processes. Thus, some authors have speculated that children are more "environmentally labile" than adults and that brief, environmental stressor-driven depressions may be quite common, but qualitatively different from persistent depressions, in terms of severity, comorbidity, and likely treatment response. Although this issue might be usefully explored, to date little has been systematically studied. A nosology of trajectories might aid our efforts to develop a sensible classification system (e.g., early vs. late onset, intermittent vs. persistent vs. single episode, or brief vs. long duration, etc.), and it might be further refined to characterize many different presumed sources of influence on children's eventual outcomes, such as whether a childhood condition seems to lead without interruption to a similar condition in adulthood, whether it exerts effects on adult mental health or likelihood of developing a disorder in adult life (i.e., as a secondary consequence), or whether it appears to evolve into a qualitatively different condition as the child moves into adulthood.

With these conceptual tools—comparing cases not just on phenotype, but also more broadly on environtype and trajectory type—

further development of our etiological and process-based understanding should become possible. Quite possibly, disorders may be classified and compared, based not just on symptoms, but also on other characteristics that might convey etiological or treatment-relevant information. Just as various forms of lung disease are classified by environmental factors (pneumococcal pneumonia, asbestosis), sometimes with implications for etiological understanding or treatment, advances in research should allow mental disorders to be similarly classified for etiological, prognostic, or treatment purposes.

To allow meaningful description, and to permit linking interventions to observable outcomes, a diagnostic scheme for child and adolescent psychiatry must capture four elements. The first element is symptomatology. The second element is development, as symptoms have different significance at different stages of development. The third element is adaptation, as many behaviors that are criteria for diagnoses arise from the child's adaptation to his or her relationships and his or her situation. The fourth element is the context in which the child or adolescent is growing. This is particularly important for very young children, who are more or less at the mercy of their caregivers.

A future DSM might go beyond phenomenological description of symptoms to include links to evidence-based treatments, pointing to symptomatic indications for treatment. This would better satisfy the indication for "caseness" based on medical necessity and the need for treatment.

For each DSM-IV diagnosis, a brief, generic statement appears about "Specific Cultural Features." In a future DSM, a cultural axis might guide the diagnostician to think less stereotypically about patients' culture, and instead to think more analytically about critical issues that all cultures address, but that different cultures address differently. Examples of these issues include individualism versus collective interests, personal autonomy versus interpersonal connectedness, the role of parental authority, gender expectations (e.g., Gilligan, 1982), and accepted ranges of expression of romantic love, patriotism, religious faith, and aggression.

A future DSM for children and adolescents, building on the model presented by the DC: 0–3 (Zero to Three, 1994), would allow a fuller description of disturbances that are embedded within the child's earliest attachment relationships, other than extracting symptoms of those disturbances and attaching them to other DSM diagnoses. This would balance the rapidly developing information in the field of biological psychiatry with the enlarging body of information about the influence of social context on individuals' adaptation. It would allow the diagnostician to capture meaningful information about how symptoms may adaptive and to make use of those symptoms as indicators of meaningful treatment outcomes. Such a model could be incorporated into the DSM as a Relationship Axis (similar to the DC: 0–3) or as a new subsection within the description of the diagnosis. This new material could be added to the current subsections (Diagnostic Features, Associated Features and Disorders, Differential Diagnosis) for each diagnosis.

Drawing from an examination of the evolutionary adaptiveness of self-regulation and behaviors, including those that generate criteria for a DSM diagnosis, we envision a future DSM that better serves clinicians treating children and adolescents because it does not constrain considerations of the child's development, his or her relationships, and the dialectical relationship among the complex systems (Hinde, 1989) in which his or her experience shapes the development of the child's brain.

REFERENCES

Alarcon RD (1995) Culture and psychiatric diagnosis: Impact on DSM-IV and ICD-10. *Psychiatr Clin North Am*, 18:449–465.

Angold A, Costello J, & Erkandi A (1999a) Comorbidity. *J Child Psychol Psychiatry*, 40(1):57–87.

Angold A, Costello EJ, Farmer EMZ, Burns BJ, & Erkanli A (1999b) Impaired but undiagnosed. *J Am Acad Child Adolesc Psychiatry*, 38:129–137.

Arnold SE (1999) Neurodevelopmental abnormalities in schizophrenia: Insights from neuropathology. *Dev Psychopathol*, 11(3):439–456.

Baker BL, McIntyre LL, Blacher J, Crnic K, Edelbrock C, & Low C (2003) Pre-school children with and without developmental delay: Behaviour problems and parenting stress over time. *J Intellect Disabil Res*, 47(Pt 4–5):217–230.

Biederman J, Faraone S, Milberger S, Guite J, Mick E, Chen L, Mennin Marrs A, Ouelette C, Moore P, Spencer T, Norman D, Wilens T, & Kraus Perrin J (1996) A prospective 4-year follow-up study of attention–deficit hyperactivity and related disorders. *Arch Gen Psychiatry*, 53(5):437–446.

Bird HR, Davies M, Fisher P, Narrow WE, Jensen PS, Hoven C, Cohen P, & Dulcan MK (2000) How specific is specific impairment? *J Am Acad Child Adolesc Psychiatry*, 39(9):1182–1189.

Caron C & Rutter M (1991) Comorbidity and child psychopathology: Concepts, issues and research strategies, *J Child Psychol Psychiatry*, 32(7):1063–1080.

Conners CK, Epstein JN, March JS, Angold A, Wells KC, Klaric J, Swanson JM, Arnold LE, Abikoff HB, Elliott GR, Greenhill LL, Hechtman L, Hinshaw SP, Hoza B, Jensen PS, Kraemer HC, Newcorn JH, Pelham WE, Severe JB, Vitiello B, & Wigal T (2001) Multimodal treatment of ADHD in the MTA: An alternative outcome analysis. *J Am Acad Child Adolesc Psychiatry*, 40(2):159–167.

Courchesne E (2002) Abnormal early brain development in autism. *Mol Psychiatry*, 7(Suppl. 2):S21–S23.

Edelbrock C, Crnic K, & Bohnert A (1999) Interviewing as communication: An alternative way of administering the Diagnostic Interview Schedule for Children. *J Abnorm Child Psychol*, 27(6):447–453.

Eisenberg L (1995) *Doing away with the illusion of homogeneity: Medical progress through disease identification.* First Leo Kanner Lecture. Baltimore: Johns Hopkins Hospital, Division of Child and Adolescent Psychiatry.

Emde RN & Robinson J (2002) Guiding principles for a theory of early intervention: A developmental-psychoanalytic perspective. In JP Shonkoff & SJ Meisels (Eds.), *Handbook of early childhood intervention* (pp. 160–178). New York: Cambridge University Press.

Faraone S, Biederman J, Jetton J, & Tsuang M (1997) Attention deficit disorder and conduct disorder: Longitudinal evidence for a familial subtype. *Psychol Med*, 27:291–300.

Ferdinand RF & Verhulst FC (1995) Psychopathology from adolescence into young adulthood: An 8-year follow-up study. *Am J Psychiatry*, 152:1586–1594.

Fisher SE, Francks C, Marlow AJ, MacPhie IL, Newbury DF, Cardon LR, Ishikawa-Brush Y, Richardson AJ, Talcott JB, Gayan J, Olson RK, Pennington BF, Smith SD, DeFries JC, Stein JF, & Monaco AP (2002) Independent genome-wide scans identify a chromosome 18 quantitative-trait locus influencing dyslexia. *Nat Genet*, 30(1):86–91.

Fletcher JM, Morris RD, & Lyon GR (2003) Classification and definition of learning disabilities: An integrative perspective. In HL Swanson, KR Harris, & S Graham (Eds.), *Handbook of learning disabilities* (pp. 30–56). New York: Guilford Press.

Frances AJ, Pincus HA, Widiger TA, Davis WW, & First MB (1994) DSM-IV: Work in progress. In JE Mezzich, MR Jorge, IM Salloum (Eds.), *Psychiatric epidemiology: Assessment concepts and methods* (pp. 116–135). Baltimore: Johns Hopkins University Press.

Gayan J, Smith S, Cherny SS, Cardon LR, Fulker DW, Brower AM, Olson RK, Pennington BF, & DeFries JC (1999) Quantitative-trait locus for specific language and reading deficits on chromosome 6p. *Am J Hum Genet*, 64:157–164.

Gilligan C (1982) *In a different voice: Psychological theory and women's development.* Cambridge, MA: Harvard University Press.

Grigorenko EL, Wood FB, Golovyan L, Meyer M, Romano C, & Pauls D (2003) Continuing the search for dyslexia genes on 6p. *Am J Med Genet,* 118B(1):89–98.

Hinde RA (1989) Relations between levels of complexity in the behavioral sciences. *J Nerv Ment Dis,* 177(11):655–667.

Hinde RA (1982) Developmental psychopathology in the context of older behavioral sciences. *Dev Psychol,* 28:1018–1029.

Howard MA, Cowell PE, Boucher J, Broks P, Mayes A, Farrant A, & Roberts N (2000) Convergent neuroanatomical and behavioural evidence of an amygdala hypothesis of autism. *Neuroreport,* 11(13):2931–2935.

Jensen PS (2001) Introduction: ADHD comorbidity and treatment outcomes in the MTA. *J Am Acad Child Adolesc Psychiatry,* 40(2):134–136.

Jensen PS & Edelbrock C (1999) Subject and interview characteristics affecting reliability of the Diagnostic Interview Schedule for Children. *J Abnorm Child Psychol,* 27(6):413–415.

Jensen PS, Hinshaw SP, Kraemer HC, Lenora N, Newcorn JH, Abikoff HB, March JS, Arnold LE, Cantwell DP, Conners CK, Elliott GR, Greenhill LL, Hechtman L, Hoza B, Pelham WE, Severe JB, Swanson JM, Wells KC, Wigal T, & Vitiello B (2001) ADHD comorbidity findings from the MTA study: Comparing comorbid subgroups. *J Am Acad Child Adolesc Psychiatry,* 40(2):147–158.

Jensen PS, Rubio-Stipec M, Canino G, Bird HR, Dulcan MK, Schwab-Stone ME, & Lahey BB (1999a) Parent and child contributions to diagnosis of mental disorder: Are both informants always necessary? *J Am Acad Child Adolesc Psychiatry,* 38(12):1569–1579.

Jensen PS, Watanabe HK, & Richters JE (1999b) Who's up first? Testing for order effects in structured interviews using a counterbalanced experimental design. *J Abnorm Child Psychol,* 27(6):439–445.

Kates WR, Frederikse M, Mostofsky SH, Folley BS, Cooper K, Mazur-Hopkins P, Kofman O, Singer HS, Denkla MB, Pearlson GD, & Kaufman WE (2002) MRI parcellation of the frontal lobe in boys with attention deficit hyperactivity disorder or Tourette syndrome. *Psychiatry Res,* 116(1–2):68–81.

Keefe RSE (1995) The contribution of neuropsychology to psychiatry. *Am J Psychiatry,* 152:6–15.

Kendler KS, Heath AC, Martin NG, & Eaves LJ (1987) Symptoms of anxiety and symptoms of depression. Same genes, different environments? *Arch Gen Psychiatry,* 122:451–457.

Kendler KS, & Gardner CO Jr. (1998) Boundaries of major depression: An evaluation of DSM-IV criteria. *Am J Psychiatry,* 155:172–177.

Kettlewell HB (1956) A resume of investigations on the evolution of melanism in the Lepidoptera. *Proc R Soc,* B-145:297–303.

Knopik VS, Smith SD, Cardon L, Pennington B, Gayan J, Olson RK, &

DeFries JC (2002) Differential genetic etiology of reading component processes as a function of IQ. *Behav Genet*, 32(3):181–198.

Lavigne JV, Arend R, Rosenbaum D, Binns HJ, Christoffel KK, & Gibbons RD (1998) Psychiatric disorders with onset in the preschool years: II. Correlates and predictors of stable case status. *J Am Acad Child Adolesc Psychiatry*, 37:1255–1261.

Leckman JF, Yeh CB, & Cohen DJ (2001) Tic disorders: When habit forming neural systems form habits of their own? *Zhonghua Yi Xue Za Zhi* (Taipei), 64(12):669–692.

Lewinsohn P, Rohde P, & Seeley J (1995) Adolescent psychopathology: III. The clinical consequences of comorbidity. *J Am Acad Child Adolesc Psychiatry*, 34(4):510–519.

McConaughy S & Achenbach T (1994) Comorbidities of empirically based syndromes in matched general population and clinical samples, *J Child Psychol Psychiatry*, 35(6):1141–1157.

Piven J & Palmer P (1999) Psychiatric disorder and the broad autism phenotype: Evidence from a family study of multiple-incidence autism families. *Am J Psychiatry*, 156:557–563.

Robins E & Guze SB (1970) Establishment of diagnostic validity in psychiatric illness: Its application to schizophrenia. *Am J Psychiatry*, 126:983–987.

Rosa Neto P, Lou H, Cumming P, Pryds O, & Gjedde A (2002) Methylphenidate-evoked potentiation of extracellular dopamine in the brain of adolescents with premature birth: Correlation with attentional deficit. *Ann NY Acad Sci*, 965:434–439.

Sadler JZ & Hulgus YF (1994) Enriching the psychosocial context of a multiaxial nosology. In JZ Sadler, OP Wiggins, & MA Schwartz (Eds.), *Philosophical perspectives on psychiatric diagnostic classification* (pp. 261–278). Baltimore: Johns Hopkins University Press.

Shaywitz S, Escobar MD, Shaywitz BA, Fletcher JM, & Makuch R (1992) Evidence that dyslexia may represent the lower tail of a normal distribution of reading ability. *N Engl J Med*, 326:145–150.

Shaywitz SE & Shaywitz BA (2003) Neurobiological indices of dyslexia. In HL Swanson, KR Harris, & S Graham (Eds.), *Handbook of learning disabilities* (pp. 514–531). New York: Guilford Press.

Tallal P, Miller SL, Bedi G, Byma G, Wang X, Nagarajan SS, Schreiner Jenkins WM, & Merzenich MM (1996) Language comprehension in language-learning impaired children improved with acoustically modified speech. *Science*, 5:81–84.

Torrens M, Serrano D, Astals M, Pérez-Domingues G, & Martin-Santos R (2004) Diagnosing comorbid psychiatric disorders in substance abusers: Validity of the Spanish versions of the Psychiatric Research Interview for Substance and Mental Disorders and the Structured Clinical Interview for DSM-IV. *Am J Psychiatry*, 161:1231–1237.

Wells KC, Pelham WE, Kotkin RA, Hoza B, Abikoff HB, Abramowitz A, Arnold LE, Cantwell DP, Conners CK, Del Carmen R, Elliott G, Greenhill

LL, Hechtman L, Hibbs E, Hinshaw SP, Jensen PS, March JS, Swanson JM, & Schiller E (2000) Psychosocial treatment strategies in the MTA study: Rationale, methods, and critical issues in design and implementation. *J Abnorm Child Psychol*, 28(6):483–505.

Zero to Three: National Center for Infants, Toddlers and Families (1994) *Diagnostic classification of mental health and developmental disorders of infancy and early childhood (DC:0–3)*. Arlington, VA: Author.

Index